THE BEGINNER'S GUIDE TO ESSENTIAL OILS

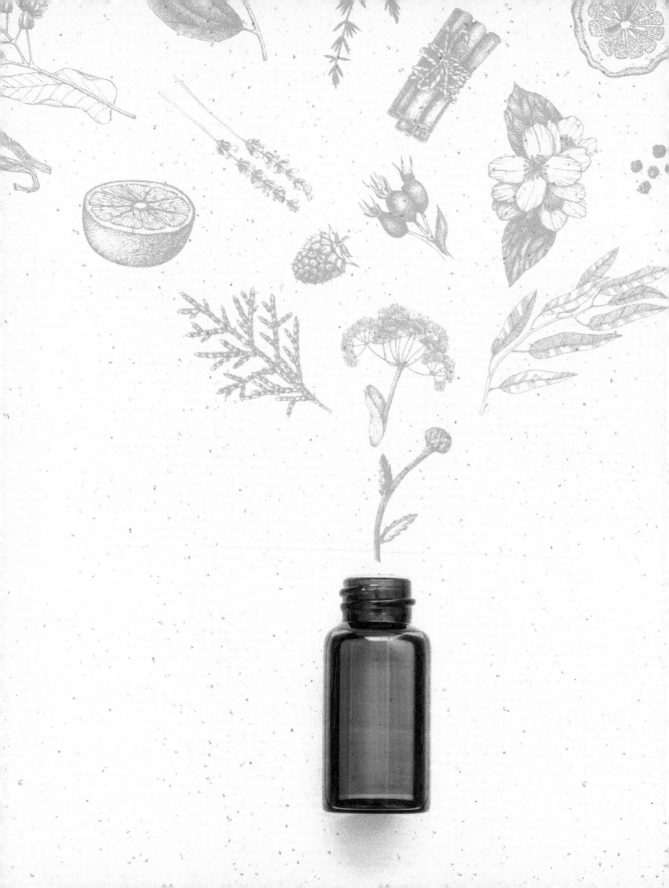

THE
BEGINNER'S
GUIDE TO
ESSENTIAL OILS

Everything You Need to Know to Get Started

Christina Anthis

ALTHEA
PRESS

For general information on our other products and services or to obtain technical support, please contact our Customer Care Department within the United States at (866) 744-2665, or outside the United States at (510) 253-0500.

Althea Press publishes its books in a variety of electronic and print formats. Some content that appears in print may not be available in electronic books, and vice versa.

Interior and Cover Designer: Emma Hall
Art Manager: Sue Bischofberger
Editor: Vanessa Ta
Production Editor: Erum Khan

Illustrations © geraria/shutterstock
Author photo © Brittany Carmichael

ISBN: Print 978-1-64152-513-8 | eBook 978-1-64152-514-5

To my biggest fan, supporter, and personal DJ.
I love you to Eris and back, Clint! ❤

Contents

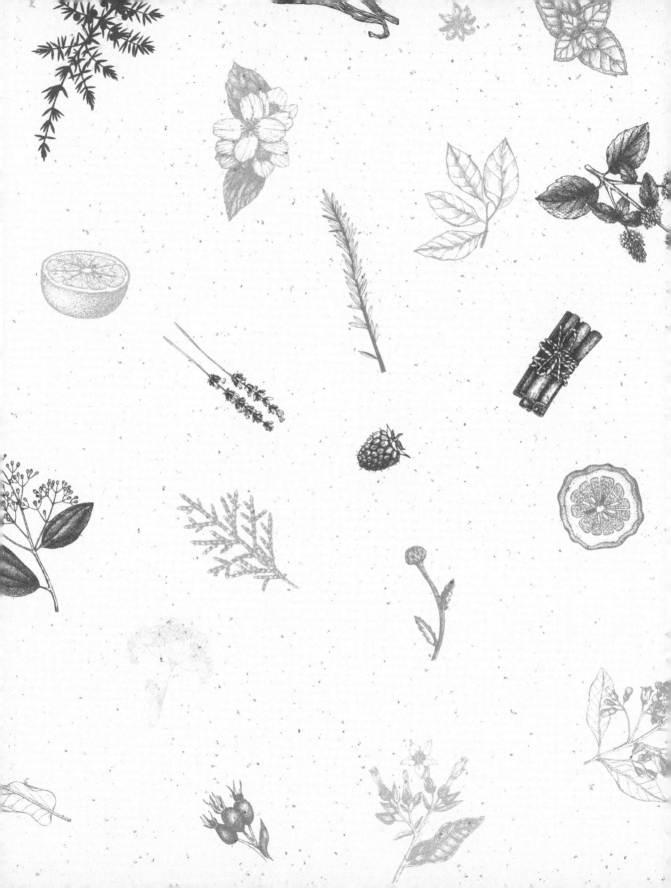

Introduction

AS A CHILD, I WAS AN OUTGOING, ADVENTUROUS GIRL who loved to dive into anything. That changed when I was diagnosed at age 10 with scoliosis and underwent a series of spinal cord surgeries. Suddenly, hospitals became my home away from home, and doctors became my teachers and friends.

Even as I grew up, my health troubles remained. I lived with near-constant nerve pain, narcolepsy, and chronic illness due to a poor immune system, and I was so focused on dealing with individual symptoms that I forgot to pay attention to my body as a whole. Finally, I decided to search for ways to break the cycle and maintain a healthier lifestyle.

My research into diet and nutrition led me down the path of herbal medicine and essential oils. The more I read about the many uses for healing plants, the more I wanted to know. Stunned by the realization that many of our modern medicines are derived from plants, I decided to take my herbal and aromatherapy education to the next level, enrolling in certification courses that taught me about the history and science of plant medicine.

I remember the first time I heard about essential oils and discovered that they were more than just pretty fragrances. Like the herbs from which they are distilled, essential oils have had a wide range of uses throughout history, from herbal medicine and natural beauty products to housecleaning and garden pest control.

Over time, I also witnessed dramatic improvements in my family's health when I used essential oils. Seasonal colds, sinus infections, allergies, and even the flu stopped visiting our home as often as they used to. And when they did show up, they rarely lasted as long as expected. We were healthier than ever, going months without illness. We all slept better, too, and my son and I saw improvements with our ADHD symptoms.

Aromatherapy, plant medicine, and essential oils made all the difference, and I am passionate about sharing this knowledge with the world on my blog—www.TheHippyHomemaker.com—and in this book.

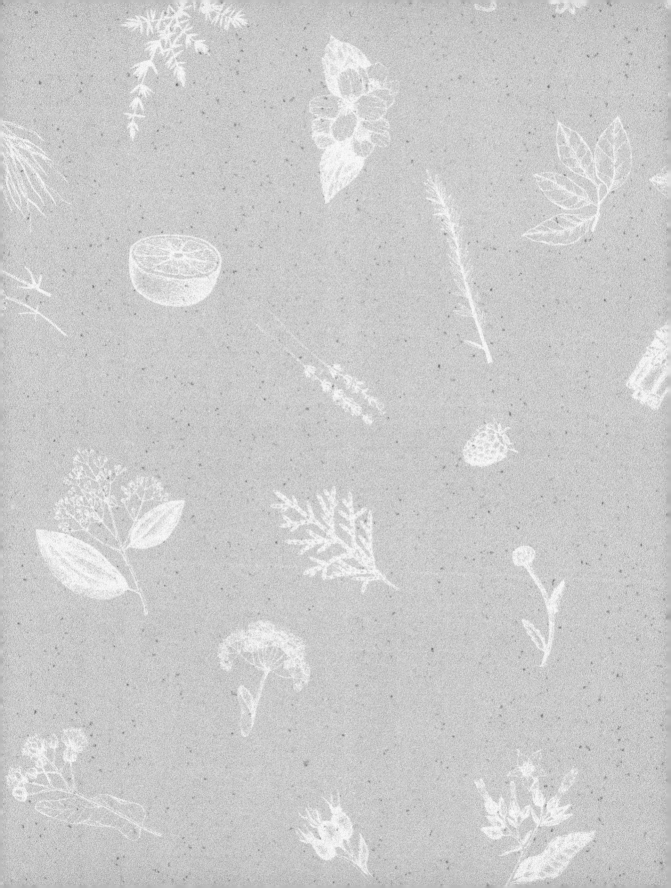

PART ONE

GETTING STARTED

Essential oils have bridged the gap between ancient medicine and modern science for centuries, and we are learning today how they are capable of more than we could have ever imagined. In this section, I'll explain how essential oils work, how you can benefit from them, and how to use them safely around your home and family. I'll also introduce you to the wonderful world of aromatherapy.

In part 2, I'll delve deeper into 30 of the most commonly used essential oils, their safety profiles, and their many uses. Finally, I'll provide 100 recipes and applications in part 3 so you can put your newfound knowledge to use.

Whether you're just beginning your journey with essential oils or you've been using them for years, I hope this book will be a valuable and easy-to-use tool in your natural health library.

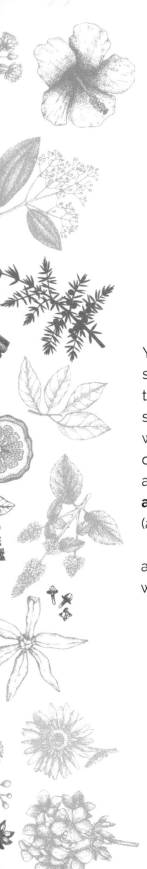

CHAPTER ONE:

Introduction to Essential Oils

You may be familiar with essential oils and their uses in spa treatments and perfumery, but did you know that they can be used for so much more? Essential oils can sterilize wounds, treat infections, clear congestion, erase wrinkles, and clean your home. Each oil has a complex combination of chemical constituents with a wide array of applications and properties that are **antibacterial**, **antifungal**, **anti-inflammatory**, digestive, **analgesic**, and **antidepressant** (among others).

There are many benefits to using essential oils, including aromatherapy, that can empower you to take your health and well-being into your own hands.

What Are Essential Oils?

Have you ever stopped to smell the roses? That subtle fragrance wafting up your nose is an essential oil at its finest. Essential oils are volatile aromatic compounds produced by plants to protect themselves, give them their distinctive scents, and aid in pollination. When inhaled, these aromatic compounds can play an important role in boosting the body's natural healing functions.

How Essential Oils Are Produced

Essential oils are produced by extracting volatile aromatic essences from flowers, leaves, grasses, fruits, roots, and trees. Some require more plant matter than others for a small amount of oil, which is why essential oil prices may vary. There are several methods to extract essential oils, depending on which part of the plant is used.

Steam Distillation. The most common method of extraction, steam distillation draws out essential oils by boiling plant matter in a sealed pot. The steam, which is a combination of essential oil and hydrosol, rises and flows through a tube into a condenser, where it cools. The essential oils floating on top of the hydrosol are skimmed and bottled.

Cold-Pressed. The cheapest and easiest method of extraction, cold-pressing is used only on citrus fruit rinds. The peels are ground or chopped and pressed or punctured to extract their water and essential oils, which separate. The essential oils are then skimmed off the surface. Proceed with caution: Due to their chemical makeup, many citrus essential oils that are cold-pressed instead of steam-distilled can cause reactions like rashes or burns on the skin (called photosensitization) when exposed to sunlight.

Absolutes and CO_2 Extracts. Solvent extraction is used when plant matter is too fragile to withstand distillation. Because it uses less of the plant, solvent extraction often is used to create the more affordable essential oils of delicate flowers such as jasmine and rose. If you can't afford the more expensive oils, absolute versions work just as well and have many of the same healing properties as steam-distilled essential oils.

Essential Oil Use Throughout the Years

It may seem like essential oils are a modern health fad, but they've been around for centuries. Research shows that the use of scented oils dates back to roughly 2,500 BCE in Egypt, where they were used for beauty, medicine, religion, and their revolutionary embalming process.

Around the same period, Indian doctors used aromatic oils in Ayurvedic medicine, an ancient system of medicine with a heavy reliance on herb- and plant-based treatments that still is practiced in India today.

Many other ancient cultures, including the Greeks, Romans, and Chinese, recorded using aromatic oils in medicine, beauty, and home care. The Bible, too, contains references to at least 12 different essential oils, including cedarwood, frankincense, fir, cinnamon, myrrh, myrtle, and spike lavender.

During the Middle Ages, the use of essential oils spread to Europe, where the Catholic Church denounced the use of aromatic oils and herbs as "witchcraft." Many historians believe that Benedictine monks, who cultivated the first apothecary gardens, secretly kept plant medicine alive despite the threat of persecution.

Modern Use and Research

While the use of essential oils and herbs declined in the Middle Ages, most of Europe's medical texts referenced them by the 1800s, along with pharmaceuticals. It wasn't until 1910, though, that modern science really started to notice their healing properties. When renowned French perfume chemist René-Maurice Gattefossé suffered chemical burns on his hands from a lab explosion, his burns led to a potentially fatal bacterial infection called gas gangrene. Because he understood the chemical and healing properties of lavender essential oil, Gattefossé applied it to his necrotic sores and successfully treated the infection.

Gattefossé continued his research and used his knowledge of essential oils to treat wounded soldiers in World War I. When he published his book, *Aromathérapie*, in 1937, it marked the first time the word *aromatherapy* was seen in print.

Though word of essential oils spread across Europe in the early twentieth century, Western physicians didn't truly recognize their medicinal benefits until after World War II, when French physician and army surgeon Jean Valnet used them to treat his patients. Seeing their benefits firsthand, Valnet dedicated his life to the medicinal use of essential oils and authored definitive works on aromatherapy.

Since then, appreciation for essential oils and their significance has grown in modern Western medicine, and experts now believe that our ancestors may have known more about medicine than initially thought. In 1977, Robert Tisserand, one of the world's leading experts on the science and safety of essential oil use, published *The Art of Aromatherapy* and brought the use of essential oils into the public spotlight. The second edition of his book, *Essential Oil Safety*, set industry standards for the safe and practical use of essential oils and was the first published review of essential oil/drug interactions. With nearly 4,000 citations, this comprehensive book contains essential oil constituent data not currently found anywhere else.

Over the last 50 years, hundreds of studies have been performed on the healing potential of essential oils, and the world is beginning to appreciate the many benefits of using essential oils in combination with modern medicine. Several recent studies, for instance, suggest that essential oils, when used with conventional antibiotics, could help fight antibiotic resistance. The antibacterial properties of several essential oils—including oregano, thyme, eucalyptus, tea tree, cinnamon, and lavender—have been studied for their inhibiting effects on common strains of bacteria such as strep, staph, and *E. coli*, and some have yielded high rates of success.

Recent studies have proven that essential oils such as ginger, peppermint, and spearmint are highly effective at treating digestive issues in children and adults, including irritable bowel syndrome, nausea, and other gastrointestinal diseases. Research also suggests that aromatherapy can help balance our emotional health. Lavender, sweet orange, and laurel leaf essential oils have been shown to alleviate symptoms of anxiety, stress, attention deficit hyperactivity disorder (ADHD), post-traumatic stress disorder (PTSD), and depression.

Many essential oils are completely safe when used as directed, but unlike pharmaceuticals and herbal supplements, they are not yet regulated by the FDA. As the science of aromatherapy moves forward, I believe that essential oils will eventually become an integral part of modern medicine. We're merely relearning what so many before us already knew: Essential oils are powerful tools that we can use to enhance our health and our lives.

What Is Aromatherapy?

Many people assume aromatherapy is just for perfumes or massages, but those are only small pieces of its healing magic. If you're curious how smelling an essential oil can reduce stress or help you sleep better at night, you're not alone! It's a common question, and the answer starts with understanding how essential oils enter your body.

Aromatherapy involves using essential oils to promote mental health and physical well-being. It's believed to work by stimulating smell receptors in the nose, which then send messages through the nervous system to the limbic system (the part of the brain that controls emotions).

There are three ways essential oils can enter your body when used for aromatherapy. They are:

Topical. Applying essential oils to the skin is a popular method. Topical application is commonly used to heal cuts, scrapes, burns, eczema, acne, and more. It also can be used as a chest rub to soothe cough and congestion, a massage oil for muscle pains, and a soothing salve to relieve menstrual cramps as well as skin conditions and acute muscle issues. Topical application generally is the slowest way to get essential oils into your bloodstream, depending on skin thickness and to what extent they are diluted with a carrier oil to prevent side effects.

Oral. Some essential oils, including cinnamon, clove bud, peppermint, sandalwood, and eucalyptus, are considered safe for oral use. This method can be effective for digestive issues, sleep problems, and urinary tract infections, but *only* when prescribed by a qualified medical professional who is clinically certified in aromatherapy. Essential oils that are ingested can be damaging to the body if they are not taken with proper care, and their use is usually limited by medical professionals to infectious diseases that require heavy doses. Be aware that some essential oils contain harmful toxins and should never be taken internally.

Inhalation. As the fastest way to get essential oils to your brain or lungs (or both), inhalation is one of the most effective and popular aromatherapy methods. It's commonly used for respiratory tract infections, allergies, headaches, asthma, illness prevention, depression, fatigue, nausea, insomnia, nicotine withdrawal, ADHD, and PTSD.

Olfaction forms your sense of smell, which is one of the most primal senses in the human brain. What we experience as a smell happens when neurons in the nose detect molecules released by substances around us. Those molecules stimulate receptors in the neurons, which send messages to the brain and identify the smell.

Using essential oils as early as 1923, Italian researchers Giovanni Gatti and Renato Cajola demonstrated the effect of smell on the central nervous system, including respiration and blood pressure. Subsequent studies have shown that smells have instant psychological and physiological effects, influencing feelings like attraction and repulsion. Essential oils work in this same way. In fact, Realtors know that the scent of vanilla at a showing can give a potential buyer the feeling of "home."

It should be noted that essential oils are different than herbal infused oils (also known as macerated oils). An herbal infused oil is a carrier oil directly infused with plant matter that usually carries only a light, almost negligible fragrance. Essential oils, on the other hand, are highly concentrated aromatic essences distilled or cold-pressed into a volatile oil that easily evaporates. While herbal infused oils require only a small amount of the plant, essential oils require an exponentially larger quantity of plant material to create a small amount of oil. For instance, 1 drop of peppermint essential oil is considered roughly equivalent to 28 cups of peppermint tea.

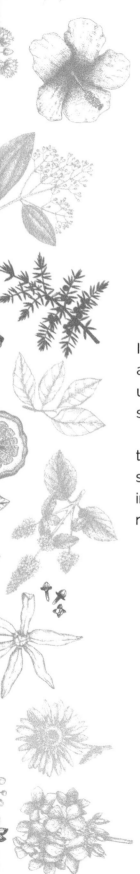

CHAPTER TWO:

How to Use Your Essential Oils

It might seem daunting at first, but you don't have to be a physician, chemist, or certified aromatherapist to effectively use essential oils. With a little guidance, anyone can learn to safely incorporate essential oils into their daily lives.

In this chapter, I'll introduce you to the basics of essential oil use. We'll cover fundamental topics such as oil quality, storage, safe practices, dilution, and applications. I've also included information on all the tools and equipment you'll need to get started on your aromatherapy journey.

Oil Quality

Essential oil quality is one of the most important topics for the budding aroma-therapist, and it can be a touchy subject in the United States because of misleading information and confusing terms, such as "Certified Pure Therapeutic Grade" or "100 Percent Pure Therapeutic Grade." It should be noted that while many essential oils are safe when used as directed, they are not regulated by the FDA. Nor is there any grading or classification system that includes "therapeutic grade," according to the Association French Normalization Organization Regulation, which sets essential oil quality standards.

When trying to find the right brand for you, here are a few key questions to ask about essential oil companies and their products:

What does the label say? The label is one of the most important features to consider when comparing essential oil brands. A quality essential oil label should contain its common name, Latin name (if it's a single oil), and ingredients (there should only be a single essential oil or a blend of essential oils listed). It also should say whether it's a pure oil or diluted with a carrier oil and include directions for use and safety informa-tion. Avoid purchasing oils from companies that do not properly label their essential oils; they could be cut with cheaper chemicals, diluted with a carrier oil, or contain a different plant species altogether.

How are their essential oils packaged? Essential oils are corrosive to most types of plastic and begin to change the moment their bottle is opened. Oxygen, sunlight, and heat can decrease their life and effectiveness. It's best to avoid purchasing brands packaged in plastic and/or transparent bottles. The best quality essential oils will come packaged in amber or blue glass bottles.

Do they sell essential oils of endangered plant species? There are quite a few companies that harvest and sell essential oils of plants that are endangered. You should research where the essential oil originates, whether it's "endangered," and if the supplier is trying to sell you an inferior/substituted product.

Do they promote unsafe use? Many American essential oil companies promote unsafe practices through their distributors, online education sites, and blogs, as well as on their product labels. To be a registered aromatherapist, certain safety rules have to be followed. Unsafe practices include ingesting and using undiluted oils. Keep in mind, too, that Raindrop Techniques, AromaTouch, and similar techniques that apply undiluted oils directly to the skin are prohibited by the Alliance of International Aromatherapists. Avoid purchasing essential oils from companies that promote these unsafe practices.

Are they overpriced or priced to market? Price can be another factor to consider when purchasing essential oils. While prices will differ, many companies, especially multi-level marketing companies, overcharge for their essential oils. It is expensive to extract essential oils through steam distillation from certain delicate flowers such as rose, jasmine, chamomile, and helichrysum. Other, more common essential oils like lavender are often sold for at least twice the price of their actual market value.

Storage

Essential oils have antibacterial and antifungal properties that prevent mold or mildew growth, but they do have a shelf life. Exposure to oxygen, light, and heat can decrease the life of your essential oils. When essential oils are exposed to any of these three things over time, their chemistry changes, and they are considered oxidized or "expired." Proper storage is the key to protecting your essential oils and maximizing their shelf life. With proper handling and storage, essential oils can last from two to five years, depending on the oil.

Keep your essential oils sealed. To avoid oxidation, always make sure that the lids on your essential oil bottles are sealed properly when not in use. Do not store essential oil bottles with glass dropper lids because they do not fully seal, and the essential oil will eventually erode the rubber top.

Keep your essential oils away from light. Essential oils should be stored in dark amber or blue colored glass bottles to protect them from UV rays. The bottles should also be kept away from light in a cabinet, lidded box, or an essential oil carrier.

Keep your essential oils cool. Store your essential oils in a cool, dark location to preserve them from the harmful effects of heat. The cooler the better. While I store my own essential oils in a cabinet, they also can be stored in the fridge. Some enthusiasts even have dedicated essential oil mini-fridges.

Practicing Safety

Essential oil safety is one of the most important topics in this entire book. Many people assume that because essential oils are natural, they do not carry risks of side effects, injuries, or adverse reactions. That is not the case. When used incorrectly, essential oils can cause skin rashes and burns, mouth and throat lesions, stomach ulcers, and liver damage. These can easily be avoided by following essential oil safety guidelines.

Dilution

Everything in essential oil safety comes down to dilution. Essential oils are highly concentrated extracts that do not dissolve in water and should not be used directly on the skin. It's important to dilute essential oils with a vegetable carrier oil before applying. You can find more in-depth information about dilution later in this chapter (see page 17).

Internal Ingestion

There's a place for ingestion in aromatherapy, but the average user should never try it at home. Just like any powerful synthetic pharmaceuticals, essential oils should be ingested only under the supervision of a certified aromatherapist and medical practitioner. Ingesting multiple drops of an essential oil on a daily basis can damage the liver, kidneys, stomach, and intestines and lead to organ failure.

Medical practitioners who favor the oral route are frequently treating infectious diseases that require heavy dosing, according to Tisserand, co-author of *Essential Oil Safety*. He says only practitioners who are "qualified to diagnose, trained to weigh risks against benefits, and have knowledge of essential oil pharmacology should prescribe essential oils for oral administration."

Phototoxicity

Some essential oils should not be used before you go out in the sun, sunbathe, or use a tanning bed. Doing so can cause a phototoxic reaction, which occurs when certain chemical elements in the oils bind to DNA in the skin and react with UV light, killing the cells and damaging tissues. In other words, if you use certain cold-pressed citrus essential oils on your skin, you may get a red rash or burn from sun exposure around the application area. It does not take a large amount of some of these essential oils to cause a reaction when used topically, while others can be used in small quantities without any issues.

PHOTOTOXIC CITRUS ESSENTIAL OILS

- Bergamot
- Bitter orange (cold-pressed)
- Clementine
- Grapefruit
- Lemon (cold-pressed)
- Lime (cold-pressed)
- Mandarin leaf

NON-PHOTOTOXIC CITRUS ESSENTIAL OILS

- Bergamot (if it is furanocoumarin-free bergamot [FCF], also known as bergapten-free)
- Lemon (steam-distilled)
- Lemon leaf (Note: This is different from lemon peel essential oil, which is simply called "lemon")
- Lime (steam-distilled)
- Mandarin
- Orange leaf
- Sweet orange
- Tangelo

Pregnancy

Essential oils have been used for years by midwives, doulas, nurses, and mothers-to-be, with research showing no harm to mother or baby. When used properly, many essential oils are safe to use during pregnancy and can help expectant mothers with difficult symptoms. Aromatherapists agree that most essential oils should be avoided during the first trimester of pregnancy, but it's safe to use them sparingly through the rest of a pregnancy following these guidelines:

Always dilute essential oils with a carrier oil before use. You should not exceed a 1 percent dilution or 9 drops of essential oil per ounce (2 tablespoons) of carrier oil. This dilution can vary depending on the specific essential oil, so be sure to check the maximum recommended dilution for each oil to avoid irritation.

Limit diffusion. The diffuser should run only for 10 to 15 minutes at a time. Pregnant women are more susceptible to essential oil overexposure, and prolonged diffuser use can result in headaches, nausea, and dizziness.

Minimize daily use as much as possible. It's best to use essential oils only when you need them.

Babies and Small Children

As in pregnancy, great care should be taken when using essential oils on and around babies and children. Essential oils should not be used on infants ages three months or younger because their skin is more sensitive and less able to handle adverse reactions than older children and adults. More caution should be taken with premature babies, avoiding all essential oil use until they are at least three months past their due date. Many (but not all) essential oils are safe to use around babies and children ages three months or older when following these guidelines:

- Slowly introduce one essential oil at a time to watch for any adverse reactions.

- Always dilute essential oils with a carrier oil before topical application. Dilution can vary depending on the specific essential oil, so check the maximum recommended dilution for each oil to avoid irritation.

  - For babies between the ages of three and six months, do not exceed a 0.1 percent dilution or 1 drop of essential oil per ounce (2 tablespoons) of carrier oil.

  - For babies between the ages of six and 24 months, do not exceed a 0.5 percent dilution or 4 or 5 drops of essential oil per ounce of carrier oil.

  - For children between the ages of two and six years, do not exceed a 1 percent dilution or 9 drops of essential oil per ounce of carrier.

  - For children six years of age and older, do not exceed a 2 percent dilution or 18 drops of essential oil per ounce of carrier oil.

- Essential oils should never be internally ingested by children under 12 years.

- Essential oils should never be used anywhere on a child's face. The vapors from the oils are too strong for babies and young children.

What You'll Need to Get Started

If you are new to aromatherapy, you'll want to have a few items on hand to easily make many of the remedies in this book. You basically need only two ingredients to get started using essential oils, but you are likely to want some other tools and equipment for all your essential oil creations.

Here's a shopping list for basic supplies, as well as other ingredients used in recipes throughout this book:

Ingredients Needed to Get Started Using Essential Oils

Essential oils. These are the most important ingredients in this book! You can easily find them online and in the grocery store. In part 2, I'll profile 30 essential oils to give you a deeper understanding of each one. I suggest reading through the profiles and selecting the ones you want to use before making any purchases.

Carrier oils. Dilution is key to safe essential oil use. The safest and easiest method of diluting essential oils for topical applications is to add them to a carrier oil. Unlike essential oils, these vegetable oils (many of which already may be in your pantry) are used to "carry" the essential oils to the skin for better absorption. You'll learn more about the most popular carrier oils and their uses in part 2 of this book.

Tools Needed to Get Started Using Essential Oils

Diffusers. A good diffuser is a must-have tool in your home. There are several different types of aromatherapy diffusers on the market, but I prefer ultrasonic diffusers, which use ultrasonic vibrations to transform essential oils into water vapor and disperse it into the air. Other types include nebulizing, evaporative, and heat diffusers. I recommend choosing one with timed on/off settings that make overexposure easy to avoid. Be sure to clean your diffuser according to its instructions; a quick wipe with a paper towel between uses can prevent citrus oils from causing any erosion.

Aromatherapy inhalers. If all you can afford are roll-on bottles and aromatherapy inhalers, you will have most of your topical and inhalation needs covered. These are inexpensive and easy to buy, and they're also discreet. You can carry them in your purse or back pocket.

Glass Roll-On Bottles (⅓-ounce). Roll-on bottles make topical application a breeze! I always keep a stash of these around my home.

Dark glass essential oil bottles. You'll always need empty essential oil bottles when mixing undiluted essential oil blends. While these can be easily purchased online, I prefer to save money (and the environment) by recycling my old essential oil bottles. Just fill the bottles with Epsom salt to remove any residue and then rinse them out.

Storage containers. You are going to need all sorts of containers to store your creations. I suggest stockpiling recycled metal tins, glass jars, spray bottles, lotion pump bottles, and empty candle jars. Don't forget to sterilize recycled materials before reusing them. I usually sterilize my containers in the dishwasher.

Glass bowls. Essential oils are caustic and can degrade plastic. I have used them to strip paint off recycled containers! So, I suggest using glass mixing bowls. Although metal bowls can be used with essential oils, avoid using metal if the recipe calls for bentonite clay, which reacts to and reduces the healing effects of the clay.

Other Ingredients

Bath salts. Baths are popular in my household, but I don't take plain, boring baths. I take baths in style, and that means lots of bath salts. It's also good to keep a big bag of pure Epsom salt on hand because it's a great source of magnesium.

Castile soap. A versatile and mild olive oil–based soap, every environmentally conscious home should have a bottle of liquid Castile soap on hand. It can be used to clean people, animals, and the home, and it's also a great carrier for essential oils used in baths.

Shea butter. While shea butter often is an optional ingredient in my recipes, I recommend adding it to essential oil recipes for skin and hair care. It's excellent in all beauty applications, and you simply can't make decadent body butter without it!

Beeswax. Beeswax often is used in cosmetic applications to harden or thicken the final product. It's needed when making salves, hair styling products, and lip balms.

Witch hazel extract. This **antiseptic** extract is derived from witch hazel tree bark and often is used as a gentler option than alcohol. Its naturally **astringent** properties make it perfect for healing skin care treatments.

Healing clays. Clays are good natural beauty staples for facial, skin, and hair care. Many different types of cosmetic clays are available, including bentonite clay, rhassoul clay, white kaolin clay, and French green clay. While you really need only one type, each clay does have unique benefits. I always keep bentonite clay and rhassoul clay on my apothecary shelves.

Applications

The three main methods of essential oil application are topical, aromatic, and internal. Note: Ingesting essential oils is not recommended without medical supervision, so I'll leave internal applications to the professionals.

Topical

Topical applications are diluted and applied directly to the skin. They're most often used to heal the skin itself, but they also can be used to target acute issues, such as muscle pain and coughs. Topical application is the slowest method of getting essential oils into the bloodstream. Some of the most commonly used forms of topical applications are:

Salves and balms. Used to heal cuts, scrapes, and abrasions, these products also can aid acute issues such as muscle pains, menstrual cramps, and growing pains.

Lotions, creams, and body butters. Add essential oils to target wrinkles, fine lines, scars, dry skin, and cellulite.

Vapor rubs. Essential oils in a vapor rub can help alleviate coughs, congestion, and stuffy noses.

Baths. Aromatic baths are used for everything from muscle pains to cold and flu symptoms. A relaxing bath with essential oils can lift a depressed mood and reduce stress.

Hot and cold compresses. In lieu of a bath, hot or cold compresses can be very helpful when body temperatures spike or you need to reduce anxiety. Compresses can also be used to clean certain wounds.

Hair care products. Essential oils can be used to lengthen, strengthen, and detoxify your hair and scalp. When added to shampoo, they can stop dandruff and repel and kill head lice.

Massage oils. Probably the oldest method of topical application, an essential oil massage can heal an injured body and calm an anxious mind.

Aromatic

As the fastest method of getting essential oils into the bloodstream, aromatic applications are inhaled and travel into your brain, lungs, and circulatory system. They can be used to treat headaches, sleeplessness, cold and flu symptoms, and to boost focus and concentration. There are many ways to smell a rose, of course, but these are some of the most commonly used aromatic applications:

Diffusion. By diffusing essential oils, you can effectively clean the air in your home while targeting any health issues.

Shower steamer. All it takes is a couple of drops of essential oil on a washcloth or in a shower steamer to enjoy a relaxing "getaway." Steam is especially helpful for respiratory issues.

Humidifier. Try adding essential oils to water in a humidifier. Just a few drops of eucalyptus, and you'll breathe easier while you sleep.

Body and room spray. Sprays can effectively disperse essential oils on your body, clothing, or furniture.

Dilution

No matter how you choose to use essential oils topically, dilution is the key to safe and effective use. Never apply an essential oil directly to the skin without using a carrier oil—also called using them "neat." Some essential oils can cause irritation if they are not sufficiently diluted. These "hot oils" produce a warming or burning sensation when applied to the skin and need to be highly diluted to prevent skin irritation. They include cinnamon, peppermint, sweet marjoram, clove bud, nutmeg, and black pepper.

It was once thought that gentler essential oils such as lavender and tea tree could be used neat, so many aromatherapists in the past had skin reactions. By using just 1 drop of any essential oil neat on the skin, you risk developing a permanent sensitization to that oil. As aromatherapist Marge Clarke warns in her book, *Essential Oils and Aromatics*, "sensitization is forever." And I know from experience how right she is. Years ago, I very unwisely used undiluted lavender on broken skin and had a reaction. Today, almost two decades later, if I come into contact with lavender in any form, I immediately develop contact dermatitis that can take months to heal.

Diluting essential oils is as easy as combining them with a carrier oil. The dilution percentage depends on the type of application, the subject, and the subject's age. Here is a basic dilution chart taught in aromatherapy classes, but please keep in mind that this is a general reference chart for blends. Some essential oils require more dilution than others, so researching each oil is recommended to prevent any unforeseen reactions.

TRADITIONAL DILUTION CHART

CARRIER OIL	0.5%	1%	1.5%	2.5%	3%	5%	10%
½ ounce	1-2 drops	3 drops	5 drops	7-8 drops	9 drops	15 drops	30 drops
1 ounce	3 drops	6 drops	9 drops	15 drops	18 drops	30 drops	60 drops
2 ounces	6 drops	12 drops	24 drops	30 drops	36 drops	60 drops	120 drops

DILUTION	USES
0.5%	Babies, frail/elderly individuals
1%	Babies, children, pregnancy/nursing, frail/elderly individuals
1.5%	Subtle aromatherapy, emotional and energetic work, pregnancy/nursing, frail/elderly individuals, face creams, lotions, exfoliants
2.5%-3%	Massage oils, general skin care, lotions, facial oils, body oils, body butter
5%	Treatment massages, acute treatment, wound healing, healing salves, body butter
10%	Muscular aches and pains, trauma injury, treatment massage, acute physical pain, salves and balms

Single Oil vs. Blends

When shopping for essential oils, you'll notice that you can purchase single oils or blends. What is the difference? And which ones are right for you?

Single oils. A single essential oil is the extract of one plant and nothing else. Each single oil is made up of its own complex combination of natural elements that work together to provide certain benefits. As you learn about aromatherapy, it's best to focus first on single oils to get a deeper understanding of their individual properties before you mix them in a blend.

Blends. Essential oil blends are a synergistic combination of two or more single essential oils for a purpose greater than and different from any one oil. Aromatherapists create unique blends to target specific needs. While you can purchase premixed essential oil blends, it can be cheaper and more effective in the long run to purchase single oils and blend recipes to suit your own needs. All the recipes in this book are essential oil blends.

Blending

Once you get to know many of the single oils, creating blends will come naturally. You can use the 30 essential oil profiles in part 2 to learn about each oil's properties and aroma and how certain oils blend well together.

The three main strategies of creating essential oil blends are based on:

- **Aroma.** Perfumers often blend essential oils by combining scents that smell good together. The easiest way to create a blend by aroma is to pick three essential oils, including one top note, one middle note, and one base note.

  - *Top Notes.* Top notes are aromas that evaporate most quickly, usually within one to two hours. Top note essential oils include all citrus oils, basil, eucalyptus, lavender, peppermint, and spearmint.

  - *Middle Notes.* Middle notes are aromas that evaporate within two to four hours. Middle note essential oils include black pepper, chamomile, cinnamon, clary sage, clove bud, fir, geranium, rose, rosemary, sweet marjoram, tea tree, and thyme.

- *Base Notes.* Base notes are aromas that take the longest to fully evaporate, sometimes taking several days. Base notes include cedarwood, frankincense, ginger, sandalwood, vanilla, and vetiver.

- **Therapeutic Action.** This blending method bases the choice of essential oils on their potential to target an acute physical or mental issue. For instance, to make a blend to help heal and clean a wound, you'd select essential oils with antibacterial, antiseptic, and maybe analgesic (i.e., pain-relieving) properties. Using the 30 essential oil profiles in part 2, you can easily create a therapeutic blend for a specific ailment, though it may not work the same for everyone.

- **Chemistry.** This method is most often used by clinical aromatherapists who have received advance training in the chemical composition of oils, their therapeutic effects, advanced blending techniques, and safety measures. Since this is an introductory book, we won't be learning to blend using essential oil chemistry. If you want to learn more about the science and art of essential oil blending, check out *Aromatherapeutic Blending: Essential Oils in Synergy* by Jennifer Peace Rhind.

You can easily create blends for aromatic purposes and therapeutic actions to fit all your needs. I suggest starting with two essential oils, then adding more to your blends as you become more familiar with them. Consider the following questions before you get started so that you can properly tailor the blend to your needs:

What's the purpose? Defining your goal will help you select a method to create your blend. If you want a perfume or cologne, basing your blend on aroma is the best route. If you are looking to soothe sore muscles, blending based on therapeutic action is a better option.

Who will use it? The answer to this question will determine the essential oils that are safe to use and their proper dilution ratios.

Are there any safety concerns? Consider the age and health concerns of the person who will be using the blend. It's also important to consider possible interactions with medications and the risk of phototoxicity (i.e., whether the user is likely to be in the sun after using essential oils).

Substitution

One of the questions that I most often hear is, "What essential oil can I substitute for _____?" While this sometimes can be simple to answer, often it takes more than swapping out similar aromas to achieve the proper substitution. Here are three different methods you can use to choose a substitute essential oil for any recipe:

Aromatic substitutions. When you make substitutions based on similar aromas, it helps to pick essential oils from the same family. Scent families include citrus, woodsy, earthy, floral, spicy, minty, and medicinal.

Therapeutic substitutions. When choosing substitutes based on therapeutic goals, focus on essential oils with the same or similar healing properties.

Chemical similarities. Chemistry is ultimately what endows an essential oil with therapeutic properties. This is a more advanced method of substitution, and Robert Tisserand's *Essential Oil Safety* provides useful chemical profiles if you are interested in learning more.

If you don't have an essential oil listed in a recipe, feel free to find a substitute using my suggestions in the next section.

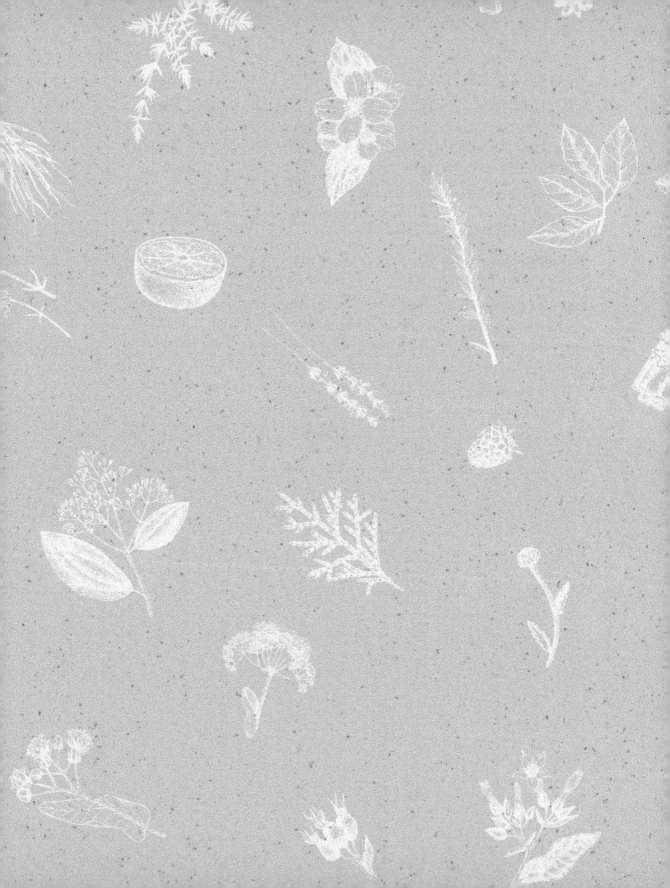

PART TWO

OIL PROFILES

Essential oils and carrier oils are at the heart of aromatherapy, and together they can create miraculous results. It's often assumed that aromatherapy involves only essential oils, but carrier oils are equally important. In part 2, we'll take a closer look at carrier oils: what they are, their importance, and their uses. In chapter 3, I'll share the top 10 cost-effective carrier oils to keep on hand and tell you about five of my favorite luxurious oils for all your skin and hair care needs. Finally, in chapter 4, you'll find 30 individual profiles of the most popular essential oils featured in this book's recipes.

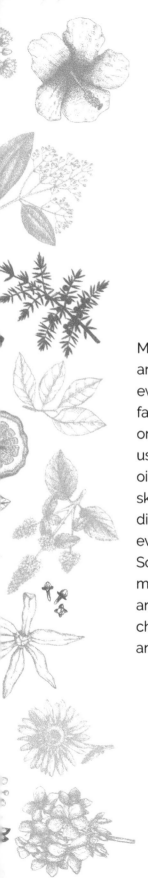

CHAPTER THREE:

Popular Carrier Oils

Many people mistake carrier oils for essential oils, but they are very different. Essential oils are volatile (meaning they evaporate) and extremely concentrated, while carrier oils are fatty vegetable oils that are cold-pressed from seeds, nuts, or kernels and used to dilute and "carry" essential oils. Often used in cosmetics for their moisturizing properties, carrier oils are rich in many of the vitamins and minerals that our skin and hair crave. All your lotions, body butters, hair conditioners, and soaps contain carrier oils. Like essential oils, every carrier oil has distinct properties that make it special. Some oils are heavier than others and are best at deep moisturizing dry skin and hair, while others are much lighter and better for balancing acne/oily skin or an oily scalp. In this chapter, you'll learn more about the most popular carrier oils and the many ways they can be used.

Apricot Kernel Oil

Pressed from the oil-rich kernels of apricots, apricot kernel oil is a light oil that is readily absorbed into the skin without leaving behind a greasy residue. This affordable oil is rich in vitamins A and E and closely resembles the skin's natural sebum.

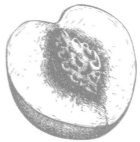

Good For: Apricot kernel oil is deeply moisturizing, making it the perfect oil to revive dry hair and skin. It can be used in facial moisturizing oils, body butters, and eye creams to smooth out wrinkles and fine lines. Apricot kernel oil also can be used as a healing oil in ointments for cuts, scrapes, and itchy, chapped skin.

Pros and Cons: While apricot kernel oil is great for dry or mature skin types, it might be too much to use alone on individuals with acne/oily skin. Dilute it with hemp seed oil to receive its benefits without clogging pores. Rich in vitamins A and E, apricot kernel oil has a comedogenic rating of 2, meaning it will not clog pores for most other people, making this a great oil for facial cleansers and moisturizers.

Safety Considerations: If you have a nut allergy, apricot kernel oil may be used instead of sweet almond oil.

Storage: Apricot kernel oil has a shelf life of one year when stored under proper conditions. For the longest shelf life, store in a dark bottle in a cool, dark location. Refrigeration is optional.

Recommendations: For dry or mature skin types, apricot kernel oil can be used in any of the recipes in this book. For a revitalizing deep conditioner, mix 1 ounce of apricot kernel oil with 5 drops of sweet orange essential oil, and apply to the ends of your hair. Cover with a shower cap and allow to sit 10 to 15 minutes. Shampoo twice, and condition as usual.

Avocado Oil

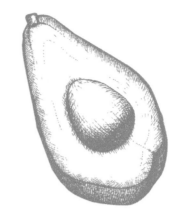

Cold-pressed from the flesh of the avocado fruit, avocado oil is a heavy carrier oil that is slow to absorb into the skin and doesn't leave a greasy residue. This very affordable oil is rich in vitamins A, B, D, and E, and beta carotene. It's also a deeply penetrating oil, making it perfectly suited to dry, mature, or sun-damaged hair and skin.

Good For: Avocado oil is best suited for regenerative and hydrating applications including eye creams, body butters, and deep hair conditioners. Added in small amounts to your favorite moisturizer, avocado oil can help smooth fine lines and wrinkles while rehydrating and improving your skin's texture.

Pros and Cons: Avocado oil is a deeply nutritive oil that works best when diluted with other, lighter carrier oils. It has a comedogenic rating of 3, meaning it may clog the pores and cause breakouts, which makes it particularly important to dilute when used on the face. Not only does avocado oil nourish and strengthen hair, but it also promotes new hair growth.

Safety Considerations: No known adverse effects have been reported.

Storage: Avocado oil has a shelf life of one to 1.5 years when stored under proper conditions. For the longest shelf life, store in a dark bottle in a cool, dark location. Refrigeration is recommended.

Recommendations: For dry or mature skin, avocado oil can be added in small amounts to facial moisturizers, face creams, and eye creams. Apply a few drops of avocado oil to the heels of your feet daily to keep them supple and smooth. For an easy hair growth conditioner, mix 1 ounce of avocado oil with 9 drops of rosemary essential oil, and apply to your hair, working from your ends up to your scalp. Cover hair with a shower cap for 10 to 15 minutes. Shampoo twice, and condition as usual.

Castor Oil

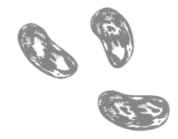

Cold-pressed from castor beans, castor oil is a thick oil that absorbs slowly and can be drying when used on its own. This affordable oil is rich in ricinoleic acid and omega-6 fatty acids, making it a fan-favorite for hair growth recipes and oil cleansing. Castor oil is great for acne/oily and mature skin types.

Good For: Castor oil makes a great addition to any hair care product, leaving hair hydrated, shiny, and smooth. This moisturizing oil is well known for its ability to stimulate hair growth, including eyelashes. Castor oil often is added to soaps, lotions, and lip balms, especially since it adds a glossy finish.

Pros and Cons: Castor oil is a relatively dry oil and works best when diluted with other carrier oils. This oil has a comedogenic rating of 1, meaning it won't clog pores and is perfectly suited to acne/oily skin types. Castor oil is the best carrier oil for promoting healthy hair growth.

Safety Considerations: Some people may experience irritation if castor oil is used undiluted with another carrier oil, so dilution is recommended for skin applications.

Storage: Castor oil has a shelf life of five years when stored under proper conditions. For the longest shelf life, store in a cool, dark location. Refrigeration is not necessary.

Recommendations: Castor oil is an ingredient in many of this book's recipes for lip, hair, and facial care. Want more luscious lashes? Using a clean mascara brush, apply castor oil to your lashes at night before bed, and watch your lashes grow to envious lengths!

Coconut Oil

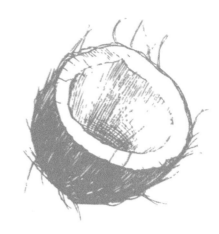

You'll come across two types of cold-pressed coconut oil in this book: unrefined and fractionated. Unrefined coconut oil has a light coconut scent, can be either solid or liquid depending on the temperature, and is a heavier oil that absorbs into the skin at an average rate. Fractionated coconut oil, on the other hand, is unscented, stays liquid no matter the temperature, and is a quickly absorbed medium oil.

Good For: Coconut oil is well known around the world for its many uses. As a highly affordable oil, it's good for all sorts of applications, including hair care products, moisturizing skin care products, and antibacterial salves and ointments. Fractionated coconut oil often is used in aroma-therapy roll-ons because it's the most affordable option.

Pros and Cons: Although purported to be a great facial moisturizer, coconut oil has a comedogenic rating of 4, meaning it will clog pores. It's a great moisturizer for the rest of your body and hair, but avoid using it in any facial care recipes. Unrefined coconut oil is so versatile that it can be used as an all-in-one skin moisturizer, lip balm, and antibacterial ointment.

Safety Considerations: Anyone allergic to coconut should avoid using this oil.

Storage: Coconut oil has a shelf life of two to four years when stored under proper conditions. For the longest shelf life, store in a cool, dark location. Refrigeration is not necessary. While fractionated coconut oil stays liquid at all temperatures, unrefined coconut oil solidifies when temperatures fall below 76 degrees Fahrenheit, but can easily be melted by warming it between your hands.

Recommendations: Unrefined coconut oil is the oil that I use most often in this book's salve recipes, while fractionated coconut oil is most often used in the aromatherapy roll-on recipes. If dry skin bothers you in cold weather, you'll understand why unrefined coconut oil is one of the main ingredients in the whipped body butter recipe. It's perfect for winter!

Grapeseed Oil

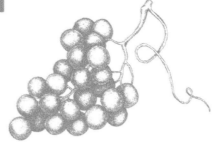

Cold-pressed from the grapeseed, grapeseed oil is a very light oil that quickly absorbs with no oily residue. This affordable oil is odorless and is one of the lightest carrier oils available.

Good For: Rich in vitamin E, grapeseed oil is my favorite for perfume applications because it tends to hold the scent longer than other carrier oils. Rich in antioxidants, it's often used in mature skin applications, smoothing wrinkles and fine lines while tightening and toning the skin.

Pros and Cons: Grapeseed oil is great for all skin types, but it's especially effective for acne/oily skin. It has a comedogenic rating of 1, meaning it won't clog pores. Easily absorbed, grapeseed oil is the perfect carrier oil for massages, skin care, and perfumes.

Safety Considerations: No known adverse effects have been reported.

Storage: Grapeseed oil has a shelf life of one year when stored under proper conditions. For the longest shelf life, store in a cool, dark location. Refrigeration is not necessary.

Recommendations: Grapeseed oil serves as a wonderful carrier oil for any application in this book, especially for balancing oily skin and healing blemishes. For a simple daily moisturizer tailored to acne/oily skin types, mix 1 ounce of grapeseed oil with 3 drops of lemon essential oil and 3 drops of lavender essential oil. Rub 3 to 5 drops of the moisturizer between your palms, and gently apply to a clean face.

Hemp Seed Oil

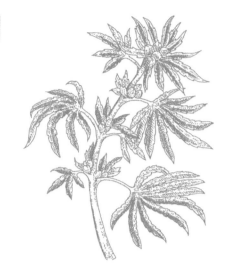

Cold-pressed from hemp seeds, this light, nourishing oil is quick to absorb into the skin, leaving no oily residue. Hemp seed oil is very moisturizing to skin and hair and suitable for all skin types. This green, nutty-scented carrier oil also is one of the most nutritive, all-around carrier oils.

Good For: Hemp seed oil is my favorite carrier oil. It's the perfect base oil in facial moisturizers, body butters, and lotions. While this oil is great for all skin types, it's important to note that it's the best choice for acne/oily skin types. Hemp oil is a wonderful oil to use in deep conditioning hair treatments because it will calm scalp inflammation, balance an oily scalp, promote hair growth, and leave your hair silky and soft.

Pros and Cons: There are no disadvantages to using hemp seed oil. It's great for all skin types, including both acne/oily skin and dry skin. It has a comedogenic rating of 0, meaning it won't clog pores and is easily absorbed, making it a great oil for massages and carrier oil in aromatherapy applications.

Safety Considerations: No known adverse effects have been reported.

Storage: Hemp seed oil has a shelf life of one year when stored under proper conditions. For the longest shelf life, store in a cool, dark location. Refrigeration is recommended.

Recommendations: Hemp seed oil is used often in this book for facial, skin, and hair care recipes. It can easily be used alone or combined with more luxurious oils to moisturize skin and hair without feeling greasy. Do you clean your face with oil? Hemp seed oil works extremely well by itself or when combined with castor oil as a natural facial cleanser for all skin types. Mix 1 ounce (2 tablespoons) of hemp seed oil with 3 drops of coriander, 3 drops of grapefruit, and 3 drops of lavender essential oils. Apply the oil to a dry face, massaging in problem areas. Rinse your face using warm water and a clean washcloth. Don't forget to follow up with a toner and moisturizer (see chapter 8, page 121, for the recipes).

Jojoba Oil

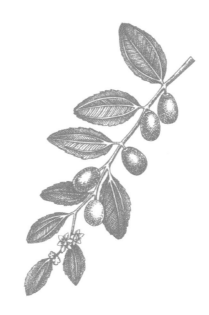

Cold-pressed from the seed of the jojoba plant, this oil isn't oil at all but a liquid wax that absorbs into the skin at an average rate without leaving a greasy residue. Known for having a chemical composition that most closely resembles the sebum in human skin, jojoba oil often is used for acne/oily skin types but will benefit all skin types.

Good For: Jojoba oil often can be found in facial, skin, and hair care products. It's a nourishing oil that works for acne/oily skin types because of its gentle ability to dissolve dirt and oil without leaving any residue. Jojoba oil is a wonderful addition to lotions, body butters, and facial moisturizers.

Pros and Cons: While jojoba oil is a great carrier oil for aromatherapy applications, it tends to be more expensive than other carrier oils. I recommend using this oil as a luxury addition to your skin care regimen. It has a comedogenic rating of 2, meaning it may clog pores.

Safety Considerations: No known adverse effects have been reported.

Storage: Jojoba oil has a shelf life of five years when stored under proper conditions. For the longest shelf life, store in a cool, dark location. Refrigeration is not necessary.

Recommendations: Jojoba oil can be used on skin, hair, and nails either by itself or combined with another carrier oil. For a fun gathering, host a mud mask and mimosa party, and feature this DIY face mask for all your friends to try:

1. Mix 5 drops of jojoba oil, 2 tablespoons of rhassoul clay, and 3 drops of ylang-ylang essential oil in a small glass bowl.

2. Add a small amount of water to activate the clay, mixing until it reaches the consistency of pudding.

3. Apply your detoxifying mud mask, and enjoy your mimosas, for 15 to 20 minutes before rinsing.

4. Follow up with a toner and moisturizer (see page 130 for toner recipe).

Olive Oil

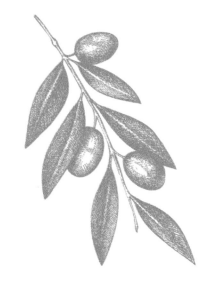

Cold-pressed from olive pits, this heavy, nutritive oil absorbs into the skin at an average rate and leaves a slightly greasy residue. Used for centuries by the Greeks for everything from skin healing to moisturizing, olive oil is a very affordable oil that can be used with (or as a substitute for) coconut oil in all your healing salves.

Good For: Olive oil is a versatile and moisturizing oil. It's the perfect base oil for healing salves, body butters, shaving creams, and hair conditioners. It has a decent amount of slickness, making it perfect for aromatherapeutic massages.

Pros and Cons: Olive oil is readily available at various prices. It's a valuable oil used in cooking, herbal remedies, and around the home. With a comedogenic rating of 2, olive oil may clog pores in people with acne/oily skin types and should be diluted with a lighter carrier oil when used on the face.

Safety Considerations: To experience the greatest benefits from olive oil, use only extra virgin olive oil for your natural beauty needs. Refined olive oil may contain chemicals leftover from the refining process.

Storage: Olive oil has a shelf life of two years when stored under proper conditions. For the longest shelf life, store in a cool, dark location. Refrigeration is not necessary.

Recommendations: While olive oil often is a go-to oil for healing ointments and salves in this book, it also makes a great moisturizing addition to body butters, eye creams, and sugar/salt scrubs. For the closest shave possible, it's important that you prepare the skin by exfoliating first. To whip up a quick and easy sugar scrub, mix ¼ cup of olive oil, 1 cup of sugar, and 25 drops of grapefruit essential oil. Use the scrub for smooth skin before shaving.

Pumpkin Seed Oil

Cold-pressed from pumpkin seeds, this vitamin-rich oil absorbs into the skin at a slow rate and leaves no greasy residue. Pumpkin seed oil often is used when cooking, but its potent skin healing qualities are gaining popularity in the beauty world. Rich in omega-3 fatty acids and vitamins A, C, and E, it's perfect for dry and mature skin types.

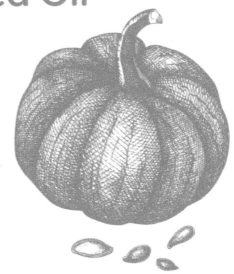

Good For: Pumpkin seed oil is a rich moisturizing oil that works best combined with other carrier oils. It's often used in skin care products for mature and aging skin because of its antioxidant properties, which make it effective at banishing stretch marks, scars, and wrinkles. This oil also is a luxurious addition to body butters, facial moisturizers, and deep conditioning hair treatments.

Pros and Cons: Pumpkin seed oil tends to be pricier than some other carrier oils and must be refrigerated. While it's great for dry and mature skin types, it's beneficial for all skin types. With a comedogenic rating of 2, this oil may clog pores in acne/oily skin types when not diluted with another oil.

Safety Considerations: No known adverse effects have been reported.

Storage: Pumpkin seed oil has a shelf life of one year when stored under proper conditions. For the longest shelf life, store in your refrigerator.

Recommendations: Pumpkin seed oil is a luxurious addition to any skin, lip, and hair care recipe in this book. Great at smoothing and moisturizing hair while promoting healthy growth, pumpkin seed oil makes a great beard conditioner.

Sweet Almond Oil

Cold-pressed from the kernels of sweet almonds, sweet almond oil is a multi-purpose oil that absorbs into the skin at an average rate. An affordable oil that can be used alone or in combination with other carrier oils, sweet almond oil is known to boost collagen production and protect against UV rays.

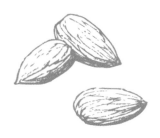

Good For: Used topically in salves, lotions, and creams, sweet almond oil can treat superficial burns, wounds, dermatitis, and eczema. It's often added to facial moisturizers, lotions, and baths because of its ability to promote smooth, youthful, blemish-free skin.

Pros and Cons: Sweet almond oil is fantastic for all skin types but may cause an allergic reaction in people allergic to tree nuts. This moisturizing oil has a comedogenic rating of 2, meaning it may clog pores in those with acne/oily skin types if it's not diluted with lighter carrier oils.

Safety Considerations: Almond oil is made with almonds, a tree nut, so individuals with nut allergies generally should take caution when using nut oils. If nut allergies are a concern, consult your physician before use. Also note that sweet almond oil should not be confused with bitter almond oil, which has toxic properties.

Storage: Almond oil has a shelf life of one year when stored under proper conditions. For the longest shelf life, store in a cool, dark location. Refrigeration is not necessary.

Recommendations: Sweet almond oil can be used by itself or combined with other carrier oils in any of this book's recipes. It's also rich in sulfur, a natural tick repellent, making this the perfect moisturizing addition to any insect repellent spray, including your dog's natural flea and tick sprays.

More Carrier Oils

The carrier oils profiled in this book aren't the only ones you can use to create custom facial, hair, and skin care products. Many of the more expensive carrier oils can be added to your mixtures to increase their potency. Here are five of my favorites:

Argan Oil: Rich in fatty acids and vitamin E, argan oil is well known for its ability to moisturize and smooth hair, skin, and nails. Known as "liquid gold," it can soothe inflamed skin while reducing the appearance of fine lines and wrinkles.

Evening Primrose Oil: Traditionally referred to as the "King's Cure-All" due to its wide range of healing properties and "majestic" benefits, evening primrose oil soothes and moisturizes hair, skin, and scalp while maintaining elasticity.

Pomegranate Seed Oil: A deeply penetrating oil, pomegranate seed oil boosts collagen production, enhances skin elasticity, and promotes the reversal of skin damage and scarring. It can be a little pricey, since it takes more than 200 pounds of pomegranate seeds to produce only 1 pound of pomegranate oil!

Rosehip Seed Oil: Rosehip seed oil is a fantastic oil for scars and stretch marks. This easily absorbed oil is rich in vitamins A, C, and E, and fatty acids, which can decrease discoloration and help stimulate collagen production. In addition to softening and moisturizing the skin, rosehip seed oil has regenerative properties that work to smooth wrinkles and fine lines, erase scars, and protect against stretch marks.

Tamanu Oil: Tamanu oil is a thick oil that absorbs into the skin slowly but provides myriad healing benefits. Known as "green gold," this luxurious oil is fantastic in both hair and skin care applications. Tamanu oil encourages longer, stronger hair, diminishes fine lines and wrinkles, and banishes cellulite.

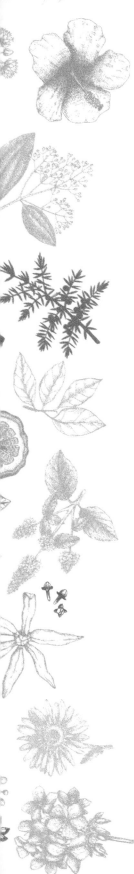

CHAPTER FOUR:

30 Essential Oils for Beginners

Essential oils are made up of a complex combination of chemical constituents that determine their functions. This means that no two oils are the same, yet they all share many of the same qualities, chemistry, and therapeutic properties. It's essential to your aromatherapy journey that you spend quality time with each oil individually to learn what they can do. While many are available, I've selected the following 30 essential oils based on their popularity, affordability, and multiple uses. As you become more familiar with each oil's properties, you'll learn how to create unique aromatherapy blends to suit your needs.

Basil

Ocimum basilicum

FRESH, GREEN, HERBACEOUS

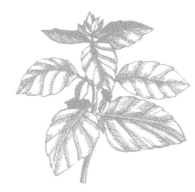

Origin: Egypt, Hungary, India, and USA

Extraction Method: The herb's leaves are steam-distilled.

Description: Basil essential oil is pale yellow to translucent and has a thin consistency. Its sweet, herbaceous, and fresh scent has balsamic and woody undertones.

Precautions: Pregnant or nursing women should consult their doctor before using basil essential oil. When used topically, a maximum dilution of 3.3 percent or 30 drops of oil per ounce (2 tablespoons) of carrier oil is recommended. Avoid use around children under two years of age. Those with epilepsy are advised to avoid use.

Uses: gas, digestion, constipation, memory, focus, mental clarity, coughs, congestion, bronchitis, emphysema, immune support, headaches, burns, bug bites, menstrual cramps, muscle pain, arthritis, energy, germicide, surface disinfectant, fevers, stress, anxiety, mood booster, water weight gain, acne/oily skin, skin clarity, oily scalp, household disinfectant

Applications: Basil essential oil often is used in topical applications, including salves and massage oils, to ease muscle spasms, menstrual cramps, arthritic pain, and gas and indigestion. When added to diffusers, aromatherapy roll-ons, or shower steams, basil can soothe stress and anxiety and help improve mental clarity, focus, and energy. Basil oil often is used in antiseptic cleaning sprays, dish soaps, and bug repellent sprays for the body and home. Mix 3 drops of basil essential oil and 5 drops of lavender essential oil with 2 ounces of bubble bath for an invigorating muscle relief bath that soothes the soul.

Therapeutic Actions: analgesic, antibacterial, antidepressant, anti-inflammatory, antimicrobial, antioxidant, **antispasmodic**, antiviral, **carminative**, digestive, **emmenagogue**, **expectorant**, **febrifuge**, **nervine**, stimulant

Blends Well With: bergamot, chamomile, coriander, eucalyptus, fir needle, ginger, grapefruit, lavender, lemon, lemongrass, rosalina, rose, spearmint, sweet marjoram, sweet orange, tea tree

Substitutes: bergamot, lavender, rosemary

Bergamot

Citrus bergamia

BRIGHT, CITRUSY, HAPPY

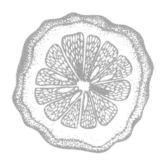

Origin: France and Italy

Extraction Method: The peels of the fruit are cold-pressed.

Description: Bergamot essential oil ranges in color from bright yellow to dark green. It has a bright, citrusy scent with fresh floral undertones.

Precautions: For topical applications, look for bergapten-free (FCF) bergamot to avoid phototoxicity with exposure to sunlight.

Uses: muscle aches and pains, arthritis, headaches, skin care, acne, itch and irritation relief, swelling, pore cleanser, hair growth stimulant, air freshener, gas, indigestion, appetite suppressant, athlete's foot, diaper rash, depression, anxiety, cuts/scrapes, eczema, psoriasis, chicken pox, surface disinfectant, cut grease, insomnia, acne/oily skin, oily scalp, improve circulation, fevers

Applications: The applications for bergamot essential oil are endless. It can be added to salves and massage oils to help relieve aching muscles, headaches, gas, and indigestion. When added to skin care products, including salves, facial cleansers, toners, and moisturizers, bergamot can help clean and treat cuts/wounds, eczema, and teenage skin conditions. Bergamot often is used in diffuser blends, aromatherapy roll-ons, and shower steams to brighten mood. Mix 5 drops of bergamot with 5 drops of coriander in your diffuser for a fresh, happy atmosphere that also kills germs and stimulates the immune system.

Therapeutic Actions: analgesic, antibacterial, antidepressant, antifungal, anti-inflammatory, antioxidant, antiseptic, antispasmodic, antiviral, aphrodisiac, appetite suppressant, astringent, carminative, digestive, **diuretic**, deodorant, expectorant, febrifuge, **sedative**

Blends Well With: basil, cedarwood, chamomile, citronella, clary sage, coriander, cypress, eucalyptus, fir needle, ginger, grapefruit, lavender, lemon, lemongrass, rosalina, rose, sweet marjoram, sweet orange, tea tree

Substitutes: coriander, grapefruit, sweet orange

Black Pepper

Piper nigrum

WARM, WOODY, SPICY

Origin: Indonesia, South India, and Sri Lanka

Extraction Method: When not quite ripe, the dried and crushed fruit is steam-distilled.

Description: Black pepper essential oil appears in shades ranging from clear to pale green with a woody, warm spice scent reminiscent of black pepper.

Precautions: none

Uses: digestive issues, dyspepsia, constipation, flatulence, nausea, loss of appetite, muscle pains and spasm, rheumatism and arthritis, tired and aching limbs, muscular stiffness, smoking cessation, fevers

Applications: Black pepper essential oil often is used in salves and muscle oils to help relieve muscle pains and spasms. When massaged into the abdomen with a carrier oil, black pepper can help with tummy troubles of all kinds. Trying to quit smoking? Studies show that inhaling black pepper essential oil in place of a cigarette can help drastically reduce the intensity of nicotine cravings. Simply add a couple of drops to a personal inhaler and breathe in its scent whenever a craving hits.

Therapeutic Actions: analgesic, antibacterial, antimicrobial, antiseptic, antispasmodic, aphrodisiac, bitter, carminative, **diaphoretic**, digestive, diuretic, febrifuge, stimulant, vasodilator

Blends Well With: bergamot, cedarwood, cinnamon, clary sage, clove bud, frankincense, geranium, lavender, lemon, rose, rosemary, sweet marjoram, sweet orange

Substitutes: ginger, oregano, sweet marjoram

Cedarwood, Atlas

Cedrus atlantica

SMOKY, BALSAMIC, WOODY

Origin: Morocco

Extraction Method: The wood and foliage, among other parts, are steam-distilled.

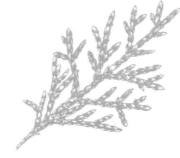

Description: Atlas cedarwood essential oil is slightly orange-yellow and has a medium viscosity. It smells of sweet balsam with deep woody undertones, like a fresh forest after rain.

Precautions: none

Uses: coughs, bronchitis, rheumatism, warts, skin rashes, allergies, insomnia, nervous tension, focus, calming, attention, phlegm, skin care, oily skin, acne, dandruff, oily scalp, insect repellent, muscle pains

Applications: Cedarwood essential oil is widely used in bug repellents and insecticide sprays. When combined with sweet orange essential oil, there isn't a bug it can't combat! (See chapter 9, page 141, for the recipes.) Cedarwood often is used in combination with lavender in diffusers and aromatherapy roll-ons to help promote calm, focus, and a relaxed mind for sleep. When diffused in an office or classroom, cedarwood essential oil has proven to increase mental focus, attentiveness, and even student test scores.

Therapeutic Actions: antifungal, anti-inflammatory, antiseptic, antispasmodic, astringent, circulatory stimulant, diuretic, emmenagogue, expectorant, insecticidal, sedative

Blends Well With: basil, bergamot, chamomile, clary sage, coriander, frankincense, geranium, grapefruit, lavender, pine, rosemary, sweet marjoram, sweet orange

Substitutes: lavender, vetiver, Virginia cedarwood

Chamomile, Roman

Anthemis nobilis,
Chamaemelum nobile

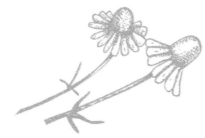

SWEET, CALMING, HERBACEOUS
APPLE-LIKE SCENT

Origin: China, France, United
Kingdom, and USA

Extraction Method: The flowering
tops are steam-distilled.

Description: Roman chamomile
is pale yellow and smells sweet and
herbaceous, like fruity apples.

Precautions: Not to be used by those
with ragweed allergies.

Uses: children's remedies, colic,
teething, insomnia, anxiety, muscle
pains, menopause, PMS, cramps,
headaches, diarrhea, indigestion,
depression, wrinkles, dry skin, acne,
dry/cracked nipples, diaper rash, earaches, fevers, infected wounds

Applications: Roman chamomile
essential oil is very gentle and can be
used in a variety of topical applications, including healing salves, skin
care and night creams, massages,
bedtime baths, nursing mama's
boobie balm, baby butt balm, compresses, and growing pain relief baths.
Chamomile also is therapeutic when
used in diffusers, shower steams,
aromatherapy roll-ons, and personal

inhalers. Are monsters in the closet
keeping the kids up at night? Add
20 drops of lavender essential oil and
20 drops of Roman chamomile essential oil to a 4-ounce spray bottle, and
fill it with water. Shake well before
use, and spray the offending areas to
calm your little one's fears for a good
night's rest.

Therapeutic Actions: analgesic,
antibacterial, anti-inflammatory,
antimicrobial, antineuralgic, antiseptic, antispasmodic, bactericidal,
carminative, digestive, emmenagogue, febrifuge, hepatic, sedative,
sudorific, **vulnerary**

Blends Well With: bergamot, clary
sage, coriander, eucalyptus, geranium,
ginger, grapefruit, lavender, lemon,
rosalina, rose, sweet marjoram, sweet
orange, tea tree

Substitutes: bergamot, clary
sage, lavender

Cinnamon Leaf

Cinnamomum verum,
Cinnamomum zeylanicum

SPICY, WARM, EARTHY

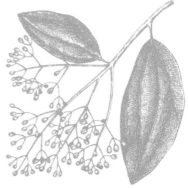

Origin: India, Southeast Asia, and Sri Lanka

Extraction Method: The leaves are steam-distilled.

Description: Cinnamon leaf essential oil has a yellow to brownish-yellow color, with a warm and spicy cinnamon scent.

Precautions: Avoid mistaking cinnamon bark and cinnamon leaf essential oils. Cinnamon bark essential oil should not be used topically. Cinnamon leaf essential oil is much less skin irritating and should be used for topical applications. To avoid skin irritation, a dilution of 0.6 percent or 5 drops of oil per ounce (2 tablespoons) of carrier oil is recommended.

Uses: rheumatism, colds, abdominal and heart pains, menstrual cramps, mouthwash, gas, pain relief, strong antibacterial agent against viruses and bacteria, respiratory conditions, dyspepsia, colitis, flatulence, nausea, vomiting, loss of appetite, chills from cold/flu, immune support

Applications: Cinnamon leaf essential oil often is used in chest rubs, diffuser blends, and antibacterial sprays around the home. Cinnamon also commonly is used in cleaning sprays to kill germs and create a homey, sweet smell. It can be added to salves to help relieve muscle pains, menstrual cramps, and gas pain. (See chapter 5, page 72, for immune support recipes.)

Therapeutic Actions: analgesic, anesthetic, antibacterial, antifungal, anti-inflammatory, antiseptic, antispasmodic, antiviral, aphrodisiac, carminative, emmenagogue, immunostimulant, insecticidal, stimulant

Blends Well With: bergamot, black pepper, clove bud, coriander, fir needle, frankincense, ginger, grapefruit, lavender, lemon, peppermint, rosemary, sweet marjoram, sweet orange

Substitutes: clove bud, ginger, oregano

Citronella

Cymbopogon winterianus

LEMONY, CITRUS, BRIGHT

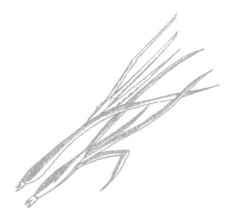

Origin: China, India, Indonesia, and Vietnam

Extraction Method: The grass is steam-distilled.

Description: Citronella essential oil is yellow to brownish yellow, with a fresh citrusy and grassy scent.

Precautions: none

Uses: arthritis and rheumatic pain, muscular pain, neuralgia, insect repellent, acne/oily skin care, eczema, dermatitis, depression, excessive perspiration, body odor, PMS symptoms, cold/flu support, menstrual cramps, fungus, clean and treat wounds, immune support, gas, coughs, congestion, lice, dandruff, fevers

Applications: Citronella essential oil is renowned for its insecticidal powers. It also can be added to salves, lotions, body sprays, and candles, among other things, to repel and kill all sorts of insects. It can be added to a breathing blend salve (or the diffuser) to help open airways or sooth a spasmodic cough. Its antifungal properties make it a great addition to fungal salves and dandruff shampoos. It's also used to help treat acne in facial care cleansers and toners.

Therapeutic Actions: analgesic, antibacterial, antidepressant, antifungal, anti-inflammatory, antimicrobial, antiseptic, antispasmodic, astringent, bactericidal, deodorant, diaphoretic, digestive, diuretic, emmenagogue, febrifuge, insecticidal, stimulant

Blends Well With: basil, bergamot, cedarwood, coriander, eucalyptus, fir needle, grapefruit, lavender, lemon, lemongrass, pine, rosalina, rosemary, sweet orange, tea tree

Substitutes: lemon eucalyptus, lemongrass, melissa (lemon balm)

Clary Sage

Salvia sclarea

FLORAL, HERBACEOUS, GROUNDING

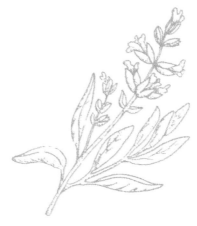

Origin: France and USA

Extraction Method: The flowering tops and leaves are steam-distilled.

Description: With a colorless to pale yellow or pale olive color, clary sage essential oil smells sweet, fruity, floral, and herbaceous.

Precautions: Not for use while pregnant, but can be used during labor and while nursing.

Uses: muscle spasms, reduce inflammation, pain reliever, menstrual cramps, PMS, childbirth, menopause, asthma, excessive sweating, oily skin, greasy hair, dandruff, anxiety, stress, depression, nervous tension, balancing hormonal emotions, nervous fatigue

Applications: Clary sage essential oil is a wonderfully relaxing essential oil that is widely used for women's health products, including menstrual cramp salves, PMS diffuser blends, and stress-balancing aromatherapy roll-ons. It can also help regulate menstrual cycles through abdominal massage. Clary sage essential oil is used in hair and skin care products and can help prevent dandruff (add 10 drops of clary sage to your shampoo and shake to blend). Whenever stress, anxiety, and hormones get the best of me, I diffuse clary sage and grapefruit essential oil around the home to calm my inner dragon.

Therapeutic Actions: antibacterial, antidepressant, antiseptic, antispasmodic, aphrodisiac, astringent, carminative, deodorant, digestive, emmenagogue, euphoric, hypotensive, nervine, sedative, vulnerary

Blends Well With: bergamot, cedarwood, chamomile, coriander, frankincense, grapefruit, lavender, lemon, rosalina, rose, sweet marjoram, sweet orange

Substitutes: chamomile, geranium, sage

Clove Bud

Syzygium aromaticum

SPICY, WARM, COMFORTING

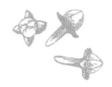

Origin: Indonesia and Sri Lanka

Extraction Method: The dried flower buds are steam-distilled.

Description: Clove bud essential oil is yellow and has a warm, spicy scent akin to cloves.

Precautions: Clove bud essential oil is a potential skin irritant and sensitizing agent. Do not use when taking MAO inhibitors, SSRIs, or anticoagulant medications. Not for topical use on children under the age of two years old. Clove bud essential oil is powerful, so a maximum dilution of 0.5 percent or 5 drops of oil per ounce (2 tablespoons) of carrier oil is recommended.

Uses: cold and flu prevention, stimulate digestion, restore appetite, relieves gas, rheumatic pain, arthritis, sprains, dental care, cavity prevention, toothaches, insect repellent, bad breath, diarrhea, pain reliever, fungal infections, inflammation, lice, poison oak, insect bites

Applications: Clove bud essential oil can be applied topically with massage, compresses, salves, and roll-ons. It also can be used through inhalation with shower steamers, diffusers, and personal inhalers and to wipe off germs from household surfaces.

Therapeutic Actions: analgesic, antibacterial, antifungal, anti-inflammatory, antimicrobial, anti-oxidant, antiseptic, antispasmodic, antiviral, carminative, expectorant, insecticide, stimulant, stomachic

Blends Well With: bergamot, cinnamon, citronella, fir needle, ginger, grapefruit, lavender, lemon, peppermint, pine, rose, rosemary, sweet orange, vanilla

Substitutes: cinnamon, oregano

Cypress

Cupressus sempervirens

WOODY, CLEAN, FRESH

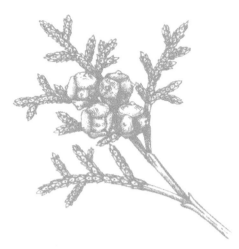

Origin: France, Morocco, and Spain

Extraction Method: The twigs and needles are steam-distilled.

Description: Cypress essential oil is a nearly translucent to pale yellow liquid that smells distinctly of cypress forests with a sweet balsamic scent with a hint of pine or juniper berry.

Precautions: none

Uses: varicose veins, hemorrhoids, heavy periods, menstrual regulation, dysmenorrhea, menstrual cramps, menopausal symptoms, severe hot flashes, coughs, bronchitis, whooping cough, acne/oily skin care, excessive perspiration, body odor, asthma, sinusitis, seasonal allergies, muscle pains, wound care, fevers, bug repellents, sleep issues, chest congestion, cold/flu care, disinfectants, masculine scents

Applications: Cypress essential oil is a powerhouse that can be used in many different applications, including topically in salves or massage oils for muscle pain, menstrual cramps, cough and congestion, and varicose veins. It can be dropped into a bath for relaxation or added to sprays and candles to help repel bugs in the backyard. When added to a facial toner or moisturizer, it can tone the skin and combat acne. Have seasonal allergies, sinusitis, or congestion hit your household? Diffuse cypress essential oil in your bedroom or in a steamy shower to help you breathe easier. Mix 10 drops of cypress essential oil and 4 drops of lemon essential oil per ounce (2 tablespoons) of carrier oil, and apply topically to the chest during allergy season to promote a healthy respiratory system.

Therapeutic Actions: analgesic, antibacterial, anti-inflammatory, antiseptic, antispasmodic, astringent, decongestant, deodorant, diuretic, emmenagogue, expectorant, febrifuge, insecticidal, sedative, styptic

Blends Well With: bergamot, cedarwood, citronella, coriander, eucalyptus, fir needle, frankincense, grapefruit, lavender, lemon, rosalina, rosemary, sweet marjoram, sweet orange, tea tree

Substitutes: fir needle, juniper berry, pine

Coriander

Coriandrum sativum

BRIGHT, SWEET, FRUITY

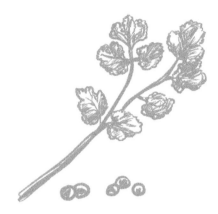

Origin: Hungary, Russia, and Ukraine

Extraction Method: The seeds are crushed and steam-distilled.

Description: Coriander essential oil has a clear to pale yellow color and a slightly sweet, spicy, and herbaceous fruit scent.

Precautions: none

Uses: stress, anxiety, mental fatigue, gas, indigestion, menstrual cramps, muscle pain, arthritis, rheumatism, depression, aphrodisiac, migraines, body odor, cut/wound care, burns, inflammation, eczema, dermatitis, fungal infections, immune support, appetite stimulation, relaxation, sleep, acne, strengthening hair, athlete's foot, ringworm, nausea, vomiting, air freshener

Applications: Coriander essential oil is an uplifting addition to any application. When added to salves, it can help clean and treat wounds, soothe skin inflammation, fight athlete's foot and ringworm, and ease menstrual cramps. Coriander essential oil can be diluted in massage oil and massaged onto the abdomen to aid in digestion and relieve gas. It can also be added to diffuser blends, aromatherapy roll-on, and shower steams to freshen a space and brighten any mood. If acne is an issue, coriander essential oil can help clean and soothe skin. For a great acne spot treatment, mix 5 drops of coriander, 3 drops of tea tree, and 3 drops of lavender essential oils in an aromatherapy roll-on bottle, and add hemp seed oil to fill. Apply the roll-on directly to breakout spots, and leave on overnight.

Therapeutic Actions: analgesic, antibacterial, antidepressant, antifungal, anti-inflammatory, anti-oxidant, antispasmodic, aphrodisiac, carminative, deodorant, digestive, fungicidal, immune support, sedative, stimulant

Blends Well With: basil, bergamot, chamomile, clary sage, eucalyptus, fir needle, ginger, grapefruit, lavender, lemon, lemongrass, rosalina, rose, rosemary, spearmint, sweet orange

Substitutes: bergamot, lavender, sweet marjoram

Eucalyptus

Eucalyptus globulus

HERBACEOUS, CAMPHOROUS, REFRESHING

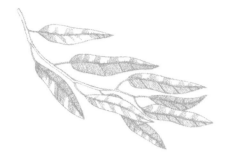

Origin: Australia, China, India, Portugal, South Africa, and Spain

Extraction Method: The leaves are steam-distilled.

Description: Eucalyptus essential oil appears in shades from clear to pale yellow and has a sweet, refreshing, camphorous smell with soft, woody undertones.

Precautions: Avoid use on babies and children under the age of six years old. The 1,8-Cineole content can cause slowness of breath in small children. Do not apply to or near the face of an infant or young child. Eucalyptus essential oil can be toxic if swallowed. In the event of accidental ingestion, call 911 or your pediatrician. Do not induce vomiting. If there are signs and symptoms of poisoning, head to the nearest medical center emergency room and be sure to bring the bottle whose contents were ingested.

Uses: depression, anxiety, air freshener, congestion, coughs, seasonal allergies, expel mucus, bronchitis, asthma, sinusitis, sore throats, cold/flu, fevers, immune support, muscle pains, arthritis, rheumatism, sprains, herpes, chicken pox, itching, acne, cut/wound care, burns, mental clarity, mental stimulation, body odor, antiseptic cleaning, bug repellent, mold and mildew cleaner, toilet bowl refresher

Applications: Eucalyptus essential oil is used in a variety of applications, but it's most popular for its use in decongestant salves known as vapor rubs. Its effectiveness in opening up airways makes it a perfect addition to diffusers, shower steams, humidifiers, and aromatherapy roll-ons for coughs, congestion, and seasonal allergies. When added to massage oil or a calming bath, eucalyptus can help soothe sore muscles, arthritic pain, and itchy, irritated skin. With its highly antiseptic nature and refreshing scent, eucalyptus is the perfect addition to all-purpose cleaning sprays, bathroom cleaners, and furniture sprays. For a refreshing antiseptic fabric and furniture spray, mix 20 drops each of eucalyptus, grapefruit, lemon, sweet orange, and coriander oils in a 4-ounce spray bottle, and add water to fill. Shake well before each use, and spray around your home on furniture, pillows, and clothing before spritzing inside the dryer to give clothes a refreshing, wrinkle-free boost.

Therapeutic Actions: analgesic, antibacterial, anticonvulsant, antidepressant, antifungal, anti-inflammatory, antimicrobial, antioxidant, antirheumatic, antiseptic, antispasmodic, **antitussive**, antiviral, decongestant, deodorant, expectorant, febrifuge, fungicidal, insecticide, sedative, stimulant, vulnerary

Blends Well With: basil, bergamot, cedarwood, chamomile, cinnamon, citronella, coriander, fir needle, grapefruit, lavender, lemon, oregano, peppermint, rosalina, spearmint, sweet marjoram, sweet orange

Substitutes: cypress, fir needle, rosalina, spearmint

Fir Needle

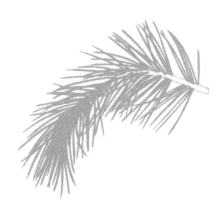

Abies balsamea, Abies sibirica

FRESH, WOODY, FOREST

Origin: Canada and Russia

Extraction Method: The twigs and needles are steam-distilled.

Description: Fir needle essential oil is pale yellow with a delightful sweet balsam and coniferous scent.

Precautions: none

Uses: eucalyptus substitute for children, coughs, colds, congestion, muscular aches and pains, pain relief, seasonal allergies, rheumatism, arthritis, catarrhal illness, respiratory conditions, wound cleaning and treatment, immune support, excess mucus, skin care, menstrual pain, menstrual regulation, fatigue, room freshening, men's cologne, cleaning the home, ringworm, athlete's foot

Applications: Fir needle essential oil can be used in a variety of applications, including as a kid-safe eucalyptus alternative in chest rubs, cough/congestion diffuser blends, and shower steams. Its antiseptic properties also make it a perfect kid-safe alternative to eucalyptus in germ-killing cleaning sprays and diffuser blends. It can be applied topically to ease muscle aches and pains in a salve or massage oil. When added to a diffuser or room spray, it freshens the air and energizes the mood. Fir needle's fresh forest scent makes it a perfect addition to men's cologne, aftershaves, and hair pomade. Is your scalp itchy, flaky, or dry? Add 5 drops of fir needle essential oil per ounce (2 tablespoons) of your favorite shampoo to combat dandruff, balance your scalp's natural oils, and bring out your hair's natural shine!

Therapeutic Actions: analgesic, antibacterial, antifungal, anti-inflammatory, antimicrobial, antiseptic, antispasmodic, antitussive, astringent, deodorant, emmenagogue, expectorant, stimulant, vulnerary

Blends Well With: basil, bergamot, cedarwood, citronella, clove bud, coriander, eucalyptus, lavender, lemon, oregano, peppermint, pine, rosalina, rosemary, spearmint, sweet marjoram, sweet orange, tea tree

Substitutes: eucalyptus, rosalina, sweet marjoram

Frankincense

Boswellia carterii

EARTHY, WOODY, SPICY

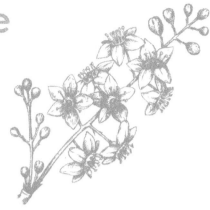

Origin: France, Oman, Saudi Arabia, Somalia, Western Ethiopia, Western India, and Yemen

Extraction Method: The gum resin is steam-distilled.

Description: Frankincense essential oil is pale yellow to pale amber with a strong odor that smells fresh and terpene-like, with earthy undertones and green lemon notes.

Precautions: none

Uses: pain relief, arthritis, respiratory conditions, asthma, bronchitis, catarrh conditions, skin care, dry skin, wrinkles, cellulite, scars, immune support, ringworm, cold/flu support, menstrual pain, insomnia, muscle pain, gas, upset stomach, nausea, acne, cut/wound care, excess mucus

Applications: Frankincense essential oil can be used in a variety of applications, including salves for muscle pain, immune support, cold and flu relief, and chest congestion. It also can be added to facial and skin care products to help improve complexion, smooth wrinkles, and treat wounds. When added to a diffuser, shower steam, or a personal inhaler, frankincense can help increase focus, relieve congestion, and boost the immune system. It's also very helpful when cleaning up the home after a family illness because of its supreme germ-killing capabilities.

Therapeutic Actions: analgesic, antifungal, anti-inflammatory, antioxidant, antiseptic, astringent, carminative, **cicatrizant**, digestive, diuretic, emmenagogue, expectorant, sedative, vulnerary

Blends Well With: bergamot, black pepper, cedarwood, chamomile, cinnamon, clary sage, coriander, fir needle, lavender, lemon, pine, rosemary, sweet marjoram, sweet orange, ylang-ylang

Substitutes: basil, lavender, tea tree

Geranium

Pelargonium x asperum,
Pelargonium graveolens

FLORAL, SWEET, FEMININE

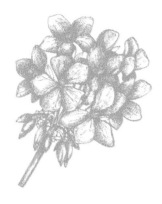

Origin: Egypt, France, Italy, and Spain

Extraction Method: The flowers and leaves are steam-distilled.

Description: Depending on its origins, the color of geranium essential oil can range from greenish olive and a darker medium yellow to dark green or brownish yellow. This viscous oil smells extremely floral and lemony with sweet herbaceous notes.

Precautions: none

Uses: cellulite, skin care, cut/wound care, antibacterial wound cleaner, diuretic, eczema, psoriasis, acne, burns, headaches, insomnia, menstrual cramps, hormonal fluctuations, menopause

Applications: Geranium essential oil is wonderfully gentle and can be used in many different applications, including antibacterial salves, skin care, lotions, and aromatherapy roll-ons. When added to a diffuser, geranium will help ease tension and stress. Whenever I go hiking in the summertime, I add geranium to my bug repellent spray to keep ticks away. (See page 111 for my favorite recipe featuring geranium essential oil, Aunt Flo's Soothing Salve.)

Therapeutic Actions: analgesic, antibacterial, antidepressant, antidiabetic, anti-inflammatory, antiseptic, anxiety, astringent, cicatrizant, deodorant, depression, diuretic, emmenagogue, hepatic, insecticide, regenerative, sedative, styptic, stress, tension

Blends Well With: bergamot, chamomile, citronella, clary sage, clove bud, cypress, ginger, grapefruit, lavender, lemon, lemongrass, peppermint, rose, sweet orange, tangerine

Substitutes: chamomile, lavender, rosalina, tea tree

Ginger

Zingiber officinale

SPICY, WARM

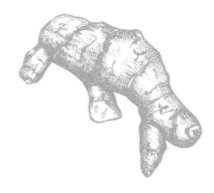

Origin: Africa, Australia, China, Germany, India, and Southeast Asia

Extraction Method: The root is either steam-distilled or CO_2-extracted.

Description: Ginger essential oil is pale yellow to light amber and has a warm, woody, spicy, sweet, and earthy scent.

Precautions: Ginger essential oil shouldn't be used on children under the age of two years. When used topically, a maximum dilution of 1 percent or 9 drops of oil per ounce (2 tablespoons) of carrier oil is recommended.

Uses: poor circulation, cold hands and feet, cardiac fatigue, angina, poor digestion, abdominal distension and flatulence, rheumatism, arthritis, muscular pain, coughs, sinusitis, sore throats, immune support, menstrual cramps

Applications: Ginger essential oil works well in topical massage applications for muscle pains, menstrual cramps, poor circulation, and digestive issues. When diffused or used through a personal inhaler, the oil can help ease nausea and soothe coughs and migraines. (See page 85 for an aromatherapy inhaler recipe for nausea featuring ginger mixed with peppermint.)

Therapeutic Actions: analgesic, antidepressant, anti-inflammatory, anti-nausea, antiseptic, antispasmodic, carminative, digestive, diuretic, expectorant, febrifuge, stimulant, stomachic, sudorific, tonic

Blends Well With: bergamot, cedarwood, chamomile, clove bud, coriander, fir needle, frankincense, grapefruit, lavender, lemon, peppermint, rosalina, rose, sweet marjoram, sweet orange, ylang-ylang

Substitutes: black pepper, cinnamon, peppermint

Grapefruit

Citrus paradisi

UPLIFTING, CITRUSY, HAPPY

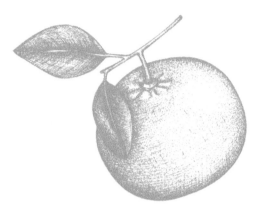

Origin: Brazil, Israel, Nigeria, USA, and West Indies

Extraction Method: The fruit peel is usually cold-pressed but also can be steam-distilled.

Description: Grapefruit essential oil can range from yellowish orange to greenish yellow. It has a fresh citrus top note that smells very bright, sweet, and tangy.

Precautions: Skin sensitization can occur when used topically if the oil has oxidized. Grapefruit essential oil is phototoxic if used at more than 4 percent dilution or 36 drops of oil per ounce (2 tablespoons) of carrier oil. If that is the case, it's recommended to stay out of the sun for 12 hours after application.

Uses: appetite suppressant, cellulite, lymphatic system booster, mood booster, stimulates digestion, acne/oily skin, anxiety, depression, cuts grease, immune support, cold and flu prevention, diuretic, detoxifies the body, hair growth stimulant, headaches, hangovers, exhaustion, stress

Applications: Grapefruit essential oil can be used in cosmetics (if 4 percent or less dilution), diffusion, massage, salves, creams, and baths, among other applications. Grapefruit oil in face washes and toners also can help with acne/oily skin.

Therapeutic Actions: antibacterial, antidepressant, antiseptic, astringent, **depurative**, digestive, disinfectant, diuretic, restorative, stimulant, tonic

Blends Well With: basil, bergamot, citronella, coriander, fir needle, geranium, lavender, lemon, rosalina, rose, rosemary, sweet orange

Substitutes: basil, bergamot, peppermint, sweet orange

Lavender

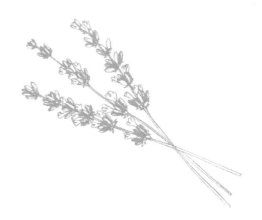

Lavandula angustifolia,
Lavandula officinalis

CALMING, RELAXING, HEALING

Origin: England, France, Tasmania, and Yugoslavia

Extraction Method: The flowering tops are steam-distilled.

Description: Lavender essential oil ranges in color from clear to pale yellow. It blends well with most oils and has a fragrant floral-herbaceous scent with balsamic, woody undertones.

Precautions: none

Uses: burns, inflammation, cut/wound care, eczema, dermatitis, fainting, headaches, flu, insomnia, hysteria, migraines, nausea, nervous tension, infections, bacterial conditions, sores, ulcers, acne, boils, asthma, rheumatism, arthritis, focus, attention, stress, anxiety, sleep issues, calming the mind, antiseptic hand soap, all-purpose cleaners, dish soap, laundry, bug repellent, garden issues, fleas, calming dogs

Applications: Lavender essential oil can be used topically or through inhalation. There are a variety of ways to use lavender, including in salves, sprays, lotions/creams, baths, personal inhalers, and diffusers. Add lavender essential oil to a diffuser to help relieve stress, anxiety, and insomnia. For a calming bedtime routine to relieve growing pains, dilute 3 to 5 drops and pour the blend into running water as you draw an unscented bubble bath.

Therapeutic Actions: analgesic, antibacterial, antidepressant, anti-inflammatory, antimicrobial, antiseptic, antispasmodic, antiviral, carminative, deodorant, insecticide, nervine, sedative, vulnerary

Blends Well With: bergamot, cedarwood, citronella, clary sage, clove bud, coriander, eucalyptus, geranium, grapefruit, helichrysum, lemon, rosalina, rose, rosemary, sweet orange, vanilla

Substitutes: chamomile, coriander, rosalina, tea tree

Lemon

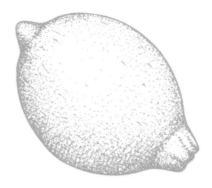

Citrus limon

BRIGHT, CITRUSY, FRUITY

Origin: Italy and USA

Extraction Method: The peels of the fruit are either cold-pressed or steam-distilled.

Description: Lemon essential oil ranges in color from clear to pale yellow and has a freshly squeezed lemon scent that is bright and zesty.

Precautions: Cold-pressed lemon essential oil can cause a phototoxic reaction in the sun when applied topically. To avoid a reaction, either use the cold-pressed lemon oil at a maximum dilution of 2 percent (18 drops per ounce of carrier oil) or use steam-distilled lemon essential oil instead. Steam-distilled lemon essential oil is not phototoxic.

Uses: stress, depression, mental clarity, fatigue, seasonal allergies, nausea, gas, upset stomach, appetite suppressant, acne/oily skin, dry chapped skin, scars, wrinkles, stretch marks, cellulite, hair care, antibacterial ointment, fungal infections, cold/flu symptoms, cut/wound care, fevers, mopping solution, wood cleaner, bug sprays, mold/mildew cleaner, toilet bowl refresher, laundry, air freshener, energy booster, germ sanitizer

Applications: The zesty fresh scent of lemon is handy for a variety of applications, including salves, soaps, shampoos, massage oils, aromatherapy inhalers, diffuser blends, cleaning products, candles, sprays, and so much more. When added to healing salves and skin care products, lemon essential oil is capable of cleaning and treating skin conditions, brightening the skin's luster, and dissolving scars. Lemon essential oil is added to diffuser blends and aromatherapy inhalers to lift the mood, banish stress, and boost energy levels. Not only that, but inhaled lemon also can help soothe seasonal allergies, open up the airways, and boost immune function. In cleaning products, it can cut grease, help remove stains, and whiten moldy grout in the bathroom.

Therapeutic Actions: analgesic, antibacterial, antidepressant, antifungal, anti-inflammatory, anti-microbial, antioxidant, antirheumatic, antiseptic, antiviral, astringent, bactericidal, bronchodilator, carminative, cicatrizant, digestive, expectorant, febrifuge, immune support, vulnerary

Blends Well With: basil, bergamot, cedarwood, chamomile, citronella, coriander, cypress, eucalyptus, fir needle, frankincense, geranium, grapefruit, lavender, oregano, rosemary, spearmint, sweet marjoram, sweet orange, tea tree

Substitutes: grapefruit, lemongrass, lime

Lemongrass

Cymbopogon flexuosus

REJUVENATING, LEMONY, GREEN

Origin: India and Sri Lanka

Extraction Method: The grass is steam-distilled.

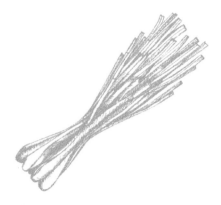

Description: A yellowish or amber-colored oil, lemongrass essential oil has a very strong citrus scent that is fresh, grassy, and herbaceous.

Precautions: Lemongrass essential oil can cause skin irritation if not diluted properly. For topical applications, a maximum of 0.7 percent dilution (6 drops of essential oil per ounce of carrier oil) is recommended to prevent irritation. Not for use by children under the age of two years. Not safe for pregnant or nursing mothers. Lemongrass essential oil also can interact with certain diabetes medications.

Uses: head colds, headaches, stomach aches, abdominal pain, rheumatic pain, acne/oily skin, deodorant, antifungal cream, antibacterial salve, insect repellents, air disinfectant, colitis, indigestion, gastroenteritis, sprains, strains, bruises, dislocations, depression, mental clarity, focus, fevers

Applications: Lemongrass essential oil can be applied topically and by inhalation. It's a good addition to antibacterial and antifungal salves, homemade deodorants, lotions/creams, and aromatherapy roll-ons. Diffuse lemongrass throughout your home to lift your mood and clean the air. The lemony-green scent that smells so delightful to us is repellent to many insects, making it the perfect addition to bug sprays and candles!

Therapeutic Actions: analgesic, antifungal, anti-inflammatory, antimicrobial, antioxidant, antiparasitic, antiseptic, antiviral, astringent, bactericidal, carminative, deodorant, digestive, febrifuge, fungicidal, insecticidal, nervine, sedative, tonic

Blends Well With: basil, bergamot, cedarwood, citronella, coriander, eucalyptus, ginger, grapefruit, lavender, lemon, rosalina, rosemary, sweet orange, tea tree

Substitutes: citronella, lemon, lemon eucalyptus

Oregano

Origanum vulgare, Origanum compactum

SPICY, MEDICINAL, HERBACEOUS

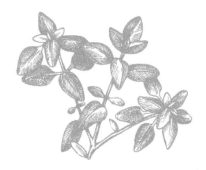

Origin: Hungary, Spain, and Turkey

Extraction Method: The flowering tops and leaves are steam-distilled.

Description: Oregano essential oil ranges from dark yellow to pale brown and has a spicy, warm, herbaceous scent with camphorous undertones.

Precautions: Avoid use if pregnant or nursing. Not safe for use on children under the age of two years. Oregano essential oil is very warming, and a maximum dilution of 1 percent or 9 drops per ounce (2 tablespoons) of carrier oil is recommended when using topically. This is not to be confused with Oregano Supplement oil, a carrier oil infused with fresh plant matter.

Uses: relaxation, muscular stiffness, stress, insomnia, restless leg syndrome, coughs, congestion, excess mucus, sore throat, cold/flu, immune support, menstrual cramps, menstrual regulation, muscle pain, arthritis, seasonal allergies, sinusitis, fungal infections, ringworm, athlete's foot, headaches, antiseptic surface cleaner, air freshener/cleaner, bathroom disinfectant, psoriasis, acne, eczema, itchy irritated skin, bug bites, bug repellent, digestion

Applications: Oregano essential oil is a very popular oil to use for sickness. It's extremely antiseptic and often is used in diffuser blends, cleaning sprays, and antibacterial hand gels to kill germs and boost the immune system. When added to salves or massage oils, oregano can help soothe sore muscles, relieve cough and congestion, relax menstrual cramps, and ease PMS symptoms. At the start of a cold, add 5 drops of oregano essential oil to a shower steamer. Relax in a hot shower, and breathe in the vapors to stimulate the immune system, relieve congestion, and shorten the length of the cold. Repeat as necessary.

Therapeutic Actions: analgesic, antibacterial, antifungal, anti-infectious, anti-inflammatory, antioxidant, antiparasitic, antiseptic, antispasmodic, antitussive, antiviral, digestive, emmenagogue, expectorant, immune support

Blends Well With: bergamot, chamomile, citronella, coriander, eucalyptus, fir needle, grapefruit, lavender, lemon, peppermint, rosalina, rosemary, sweet marjoram, sweet orange, tea tree

Substitutes: clove bud, sweet marjoram, tea tree, thyme

Peppermint

Mentha x piperita

FRESH, MINTY, COOLING

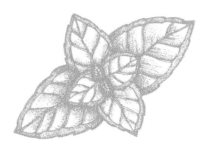

Origin: Southern Europe and USA

Extraction Method: The leaves are steam-distilled.

Description: Ranging in color from pale yellow to pale olive, peppermint essential oil is viscous and has a fresh, minty, herbal scent with balsamic-sweet undertones.

Precautions: Not for use with children under the age of six years due to the menthol and 1,8-Cineole content. Do not apply on or near the face of an infant or child. When used topically, a maximum dilution of 5 percent or 45 drops per ounce (2 tablespoons) of carrier oil is recommended.

Uses: digestive issues, colon, nausea, acid reflux, dyspepsia, stomach pains, diarrhea, flatulence, muscle pains, toothpaste, oral care, decongestant, pain relief, cooling burns, skin irritation, acne, circulation issues, headaches/migraines, cold and flu symptoms, cleaning the lymphatic system, fevers

Applications: Peppermint essential oil can be used in oral care applications, including homemade toothpaste and mouthwash. It's great for topical use in skin care salves, cooling sprays, and roll-ons. Inhalation often is used to help relieve congestion with shower steamers, diffusers, and personal inhalers.

Therapeutic Actions: analgesic, antibacterial, antifungal, anti-inflammatory, antimicrobial, antiseptic, antispasmodic, astringent, carminative, digestive, emmenagogue, expectorant, febrifuge, insecticide, nervine, sedative, stimulant, vasoconstrictor

Blends Well With: basil, black pepper, coriander, eucalyptus, fir needle, lavender, lemon, pine, rosalina, rosemary, spearmint, sweet marjoram, tea tree, thyme

Substitute: spearmint

Rosalina

Melaleuca ericifolia

FLORAL, LEMONY, MEDICINAL

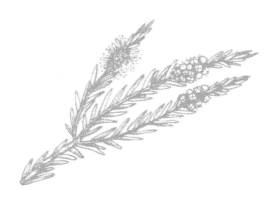

Origin: Australia

Extraction Method: The leaves are steam-distilled.

Description: Rosalina essential oil has a clear to pale yellow color and a soft, lemony, medicinal scent with floral undertones.

Precautions: none

Uses: asthma, seasonal allergies, burn relief, after-sun care, bug sprays, catarrh, coughs, congestion, expel mucus, sore throat, sniffles, sneezing, runny nose, circulation, cold/flu symptoms, ear infections, headaches, itch relief, fevers, germs, immune support, pain relief, muscle pain, menstrual cramps, warts, depression, anxiety, air freshener, chicken pox, acne, cut/wound care, mental clarity, body odor, antiseptic cleaning sprays, insomnia, stress, tension

Applications: Rosalina essential oil is a gentle, kid-safe alternative to eucalyptus and can be used in any application that calls for eucalyptus. When added to salves, massage oils, diffuser blends, and aromatherapy inhalers, rosalina essential oil can help open airways and ease coughs, congestion, and stuffy noses. It's often added to skin care products, including facial toners, moisturizers, and antibacterial "owie" creams to soothe and treat acne, dry flaky skin, cuts, and abrasions. Rosalina's insecticidal properties make it the perfect addition to lice-killing treatments as well as kid-friendly bug sprays. Does your young one have a headache? Drop 15 drops of rosalina and 10 drops of lavender essential oils into a ⅓-ounce aromatherapy roll-on bottle. Swirl to mix, and fill with a carrier oil. Roll onto the temples and back of the neck, and gently massage to relieve the pain.

Therapeutic Actions: analgesic, antibacterial, antidepressant, antifungal, anti-inflammatory, antimicrobial, antiseptic, antispasmodic, antiviral, decongestant, expectorant, febrifuge, insecticide, sedative, vulnerary

Blends Well With: bergamot, cedarwood, chamomile, cinnamon, citronella, coriander, eucalyptus, fir needle, frankincense, geranium, grapefruit, lavender, lemon, spearmint, sweet marjoram, sweet orange

Substitutes: eucalyptus, lavender, sweet marjoram, tea tree

Rose

Rosa damascena, Rose otto

FLORAL, SWEET, RICH

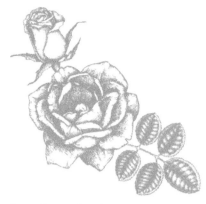

Origin: Morocco

Extraction Method: The flowers are steam-distilled. For the less expensive version, rose absolute, the flowers are solvent-extracted.

Description: Rose essential oil is orange- to brown-yellow and quite viscous. It has a sweet floral scent that smells of honey and spicy notes. Rose absolute is dark orange to red and smells heavily of roses.

Precautions: When used topically, a maximum dilution of 0.6 percent or 5 drops per ounce (2 tablespoons) of carrier oil is recommended.

Uses: cold sores, nerve sedative, insomnia, irritability, female sexual issues, uterine tonic, regulate menstruation, cramps, excessive menstrual bleeding, anxiety, irregular periods, soften skin, acne, scars, facial cleansing, wrinkles, mature skin, dry skin, sensitive skin, perfume

Applications: Rose essential oil is a gentle, healing oil found in many skin care products, including eye creams, lotions, soaps, wrinkle treatments, bath products, facial cleaning products, toners, and facial moisturizers. Rose also is used in women's menstruation salves and aromatherapy roll-ons to soothe PMS symptoms. When diffused at home and sprayed on pillows and blankets, rose essential oil provides an enduring, romantic scent.

Therapeutic Actions: analgesic, antibacterial, antidepressant, antifungal, anti-inflammatory, anti-microbial, antiseptic, antispasmodic, antiviral, aphrodisiac, astringent, bactericidal, cicatrizant, deodorant, disinfectant, diuretic, emmenagogue, nervine, sedative

Blends Well With: bergamot, black pepper, cedarwood, chamomile, coriander, geranium, grapefruit, lavender, lemon, rosalina, spearmint, sweet orange, tea tree

Substitutes: frankincense, geranium, rose absolute

Rosemary

Rosmarinus officinalis

FRESH, WOODY, CAMPHOROUS

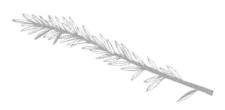

Origin: France, Greece, Italy, Spain, and Tunisia

Extraction Method: The flowering tops and leaves are steam-distilled.

Description: Rosemary essential oil has a clear to pale yellow color and a fresh herbaceous scent with medicinal woody undertones.

Precautions: Not for pregnant or nursing women. Avoid use with epilepsy. Not safe for use on children under the age of six years. Do not apply on or near the face of an infant or child. Rosemary essential oil can cause skin irritation if not properly diluted. It's recommended to use a maximum dilution of 4 percent or 36 drops per ounce (2 tablespoons) of carrier oil for topical applications.

Uses: mental clarity/energy, focus, depression, lethargy, immune support, kill germs, air freshener/cleaner, muscle pain, arthritis, rheumatism, menstrual pain, antiseptic cleaning sprays, dish soap, insect repellent, lice, dandruff, hair repair, hair growth, acne/oily skin, oily scalp, coughs, congestion, expel mucus, cold/flu, cut/wound care, burns

Applications: Rosemary essential oil can be used topically in salves and massage oils to help relieve coughs, congestion, muscle aches, and menstrual pain. When added to a diffuser, aromatherapy roll-ons, or personal inhalers, rosemary soothes seasonal allergies, increases mental focus, and kills germs. Rosemary is great for hair, balancing an oily scalp, getting rid of dandruff, and killing lice when added to shampoo. Its antibacterial and stimulating properties make rosemary a great addition to cleaners, toners, and moisturizers for acne/oily skin types. Add 1 drop of rosemary essential oil to a quart-size shampoo bottle two to three times a week for healthier, shinier, and more lustrous hair.

Therapeutic Actions: analgesic, antibacterial, antifungal, anti-inflammatory, antimicrobial, antioxidant, antirheumatic, antiseptic, antispasmodic, antitussive, antiviral, astringent, decongestant, carminative, digestive, expectorant, stimulant

Blends Well With: basil, bergamot, black pepper, cedarwood, cinnamon, citronella, clove bud, cypress, eucalyptus, fir needle, ginger, grapefruit, lavender, lemon, oregano, peppermint, rosalina, spearmint, sweet marjoram, tea tree

Substitutes: cypress, fir needle, oregano, sweet marjoram

Spearmint

Mentha spicata

MINTY, SWEET, FRESH

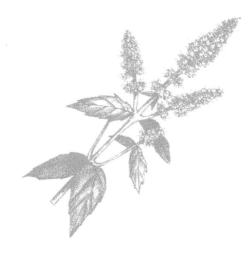

Origin: Worldwide (India and USA are the largest suppliers)

Extraction Method: The flowering tops and leaves are steam-distilled.

Description: Ranging in color from pale yellow to pale olive, spearmint essential oil has a green herbaceous scent like the crushed herb.

Precautions: When used topically, a maximum dilution of 1.7 percent or 15 drops per ounce (2 tablespoons) of carrier oil is recommended.

Uses: dental hygiene, digestion, gas, upset stomach, pain relief, fevers, sinus issues, seasonal allergies, decongestant, cleaning, kid-safe peppermint alternative, acne, dermatitis, congested skin, asthma, lift mood, mental strain, fatigue, stress, depression

Applications: Spearmint essential oil is a wonderful, kid-friendly oil that can be substituted for peppermint in chest congestion salves and seasonal allergy inhalers. When mixed with a carrier oil, spearmint essential oil can be massaged on the abdomen for gas and upset tummies or into muscles for pain relief. Spearmint may be added to a diffuser, shower steamer, or personal inhaler to help with allergies, sinus congestion, and mood. (See page 106 for a kid-safe vapor rub recipe.)

Therapeutic Actions: analgesic, anesthetic, antibacterial, anti-inflammatory, antiseptic, antispasmodic, astringent, carminative, decongestant, digestive, diuretic, emmenagogue, expectorant, febrifuge, insecticidal, nervine, stimulant

Blends Well With: basil, bergamot, cedarwood, chamomile, eucalyptus, fir needle, grapefruit, lavender, peppermint, pine, rosalina, sweet marjoram, sweet orange, tea tree

Substitutes: ginger, peppermint, rosalina

Sweet Marjoram

Majorana hortensis, Origanum majorana

FRESH, CLEAN, CAMPHOROUS

Origin: Egypt and Hungary

Extraction Method: The dried leaves and flowering tops are steam-distilled.

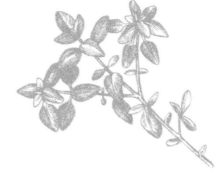

Description: Sweet marjoram essential oil is a pale yellow or pale amber oil that can be very viscous. It smells warm, spicy, camphorous, and woodsy.

Precautions: Not to be confused with Spanish Marjoram (*Thymus mastichina*).

Uses: muscular stiffness/pain, nerve spasms/pains, arthritis, intestinal colic, insomnia, restless leg syndrome, rheumatic pains, strains, sprains, tension, chest colds, coughs, congestion, antibacterial rub during cold/flu, menstrual cramps, anxiety, nervousness

Applications: Sweet marjoram essential oil can be used topically with massages, compresses, baths, salves, and skin care products. It also can be inhaled with a diffuser, shower steamer, or straight from the bottle. Add 3 to 5 drops per ounce (2 tablespoons) of your favorite bubble bath for a muscle pain–relieving bath soak.

Therapeutic Actions: analgesic, antioxidant, antiseptic, antispasmodic, antiviral, bactericidal, carminative, cephalic, diaphoretic, digestive, diuretic, emmenagogue, expectorant, fungicidal, nervine, sedative, vasodilator, vulnerary

Blends Well With: bergamot, cedarwood, chamomile, citronella, eucalyptus, fir needle, lavender, lemon, oregano, pine, rosalina, sweet orange, tea tree, thyme

Substitutes: black pepper, lavender, oregano, pine

Sweet Orange

Citrus sinensis

SWEET, CITRUSY, BRIGHT

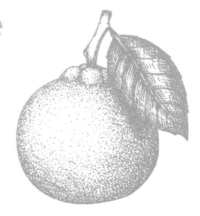

Origin: Australia, Brazil, Israel, and North America

Extraction Method: The fruit peel is usually cold-pressed but also can be steam-distilled.

Description: Sweet orange comes in different shades of orange and has a fresh citrus odor that smells like orange peels.

Precautions: none

Uses: household cleaners, upset stomach, insomnia, digestive issues, stimulate the lymphatic system, spasms, cramps, constipation, flatulence, IBS, cellulite, sedative, acne/oily skin, dry skin, depression, anxiety, nervousness

Applications: Sweet orange is a gentle essential oil commonly used for salves, skin care, facial care, baths, shower steamers, and toothpaste. It's also the perfect essential oil to clean your home because it cuts grease, removes sticky stuff off jars, and kills bugs. Diffuse sweet orange essential oil to disinfect your home and boost immune support.

Therapeutic Actions: anticoagulant, antidepressant, anti-inflammatory, antiseptic, antispasmodic, bactericidal, carminative, cholagogue, digestive, diuretic, expectorant, fungicidal, lymphatic stimulant, sedative, stimulant, stomachic, tonic

Blends Well With: basil, bergamot, black pepper, cedarwood, chamomile, cinnamon, clove bud, coriander, eucalyptus, fir needle, frankincense, ginger, grapefruit, lavender, lemon, pine, rose, rosalina, spearmint, tea tree

Substitutes: blood orange, grapefruit, mandarin, tangerine

Tea Tree

Melaleuca alternifolia

WOODY, MEDICINAL, WARM

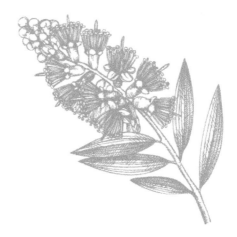

Origin: Australia, New Zealand, and USA

Extraction Method: The leaves are steam-distilled.

Description: Tea tree essential oil comes in shades that vary from clear to pale yellow. It has a refreshing, camphorous scent with green, woody undertones.

Precautions: Tea tree essential oil can be toxic if swallowed. In the event of accidental ingestion, call 911 or your pediatrician/primary care physician. Do not induce vomiting. If signs and symptoms of poisoning occur, head to a medical center emergency room with the essential oil bottle.

Uses: stress, anxiety, mental clarity, insomnia, congestion, respiratory issues, coughs, stuffy noses, cold/flu, sinusitis, fevers, seasonal allergies, cuts/scrapes, burns, sunburns, sores, bug bites, scars, acne/oily skin, eczema, dermatitis, athlete's foot, ringworm, warts, skin tags, body odor, dandruff, lice, strengthen hair, oily scalp, antiseptic cleaning sprays, disinfect bathrooms, toilet bowl cleaner, mold/mildew spray, fungus control in the garden

Applications: Tea tree essential oil has many applications, but it's most popular for its antibacterial properties. Tea tree is used in facial cleaners, toners, and moisturizers to treat wounds, acne, and oily skin. In a salve or diluted in a carrier oil, it can treat cuts, scrapes, burns, eczema, and fungal infections. It's typically diffused or inhaled through a personal inhaler to relieve cold and flu symptoms, disinfect an area, and stimulate the immune system. Add tea tree oil to a shower steamer or a personal steam bowl to help clear congestion and treat a sinus infection. Mix 30 drops of tea tree essential oil per ounce (2 tablespoons) of coconut oil, and regularly apply to dry feet after bathing to avoid foot fungus. >>

Therapeutic Actions: antibacterial, antifungal, anti-infectious, anti-inflammatory, antimicrobial, antiseptic, antiviral, cicatrizant, decongestant, disinfectant, expectorant, febrifuge, fungicide, immune stimulant, immune support, insecticidal, sedative, vulnerary

Blends Well With: bergamot, chamomile, coriander, cypress, grapefruit, lavender, lemon, oregano, peppermint, rosalina, rosemary, spearmint, sweet marjoram, sweet orange

Substitutes: geranium, lavender, rosalina

Ylang-Ylang

Cananga odorata

FLORAL, SWEET, WARM

Origin: Madagascar

Extraction Method: The flowers are steam-distilled.

Description: There are two different types of ylang-ylang essential oil: extra and complete. Ylang-ylang extra is pale yellow and has an intense floral scent that can be soft and sweet. A yellowish oily liquid, ylang-ylang complete has a sweet floral scent with a balsamic, woody base note.

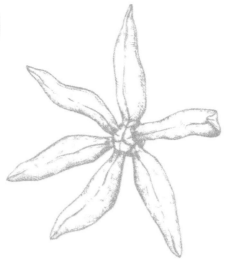

Precautions: Not for use on children under two years of age and pregnant or nursing mothers. When used topically, a maximum dermal level of 0.8 percent or 7 drops per ounce (2 tablespoons) of carrier oil is recommended.

Uses: skin conditions, cosmetics, hair care products, perfumes, depression, insomnia, muscle spasms, aphrodisiac, dry and oily skin, PMS, mood swings

Applications: Ylang-ylang essential oil is used topically in cosmetics and skin care products to help soothe and treat dry skin, smooth wrinkles, and reduce scarring. When diffused, it can ease tension, lift mood, and add a little romance to the atmosphere. Add 1 drop of ylang-ylang essential oil per ounce (2 tablespoons) of avocado oil for a luxurious facial moisturizer.

Therapeutic Actions: antibacterial, antidepressant, antifungal, anti-inflammatory, antiseptic, antispasmodic, aphrodisiac, expectorant, hypotensive, nervine, sedative, vulnerary

Blends Well With: bergamot, black pepper, cedarwood, chamomile, clary sage, clove bud, geranium, ginger, grapefruit, lavender, lemon, lemongrass, rosalina, rose, sweet orange

Substitutes: helichrysum, jasmine, patchouli

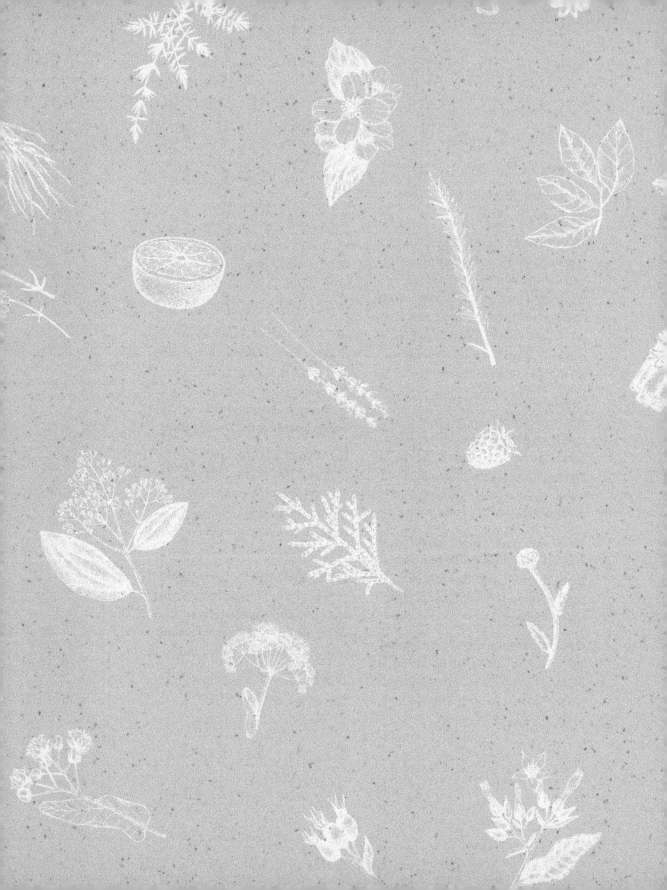

PART THREE

RECIPES AND APPLICATIONS

The benefits of essential oils are endless. They can help improve physical and mental health, enhance cosmetics and toiletries, and disinfect and clean your home. This section features 100 recipes using the essential oils to which you have been introduced. Chapter 5 is full of recipes for everything from cough and congestion to fevers, headaches, and more. Chapter 6 targets emotional health, including recipes for improved focus and energy, reduced anxiety, and appetite suppression. In chapter 7, you'll find family-specific recipes for pregnant mothers, babies and children, women, men, and older family members. Chapter 8 highlights recipes for personal care, including toothpaste, deodorant, facial care, and more. And in chapter 9, you'll learn how to make your own natural cleaning supplies for every room in your home.

CHAPTER FIVE

For Physical Health

Plague Killer Diffuser Blend

Nothing kills germs like this highly antibacterial and antiviral essential oil blend. Diffuse it in every room to disinfect your home, support the immune system, and ease cold and flu symptoms.

1. Add all the essential oils to an empty essential oil bottle (or any dark glass bottle with a dropper), and gently swirl to blend.

2. Add 8 to 10 drops to a diffuser, and diffuse in 30-minute increments (30 minutes on/ 30 minutes off).

Makes ½ ounce

¾ teaspoon eucalyptus essential oil

1 teaspoon cinnamon leaf essential oil

¼ teaspoon clove bud essential oil

¾ teaspoon lemon essential oil

¼ teaspoon rosemary essential oil

Helpful Hint: This essential oil blend can be used in any of the cleaning, shower steamer, and personal aromatherapy inhaler recipes in this book.

Citrus Fresh Antibacterial Foaming Hand Soap

This fresh-smelling foaming soap gently cleans and moisturizes hands. It's safe for the whole family to use, and making your own hand soap will save you money, too!

1. Mix all ingredients in a 250 ml (about 1 cup) foaming pump bottle. Seal the lid, and gently shake to blend.

2. Store on bathroom or kitchen sinks for easy, everyday use.

Makes 250 ml
(about 1 cup)

1 tablespoon liquid Castile soap

1 tablespoon avocado oil (or another liquid carrier oil)

5 drops sweet orange essential oil

5 drops grapefruit essential oil

5 drops bergamot essential oil

5 drops spearmint essential oil

Filtered water, to fill

Breathe Better Vapor Rub

TOPICAL

Safe for ages 6+. Not safe for pregnant or nursing mothers

When cough and congestion strike, this classic vapor rub remedy can help everyone breathe better. (See page 106 for a kid-friendly version.)

1. In a pan over low heat, melt the coconut oil and beeswax.

2. Once melted, remove from heat, and add the essential oils.

3. Pour into a 4-ounce mason jar, and put into the freezer for about 20 minutes to harden.

4. Apply to your chest, back, and neck.

Makes about 4 ounces

¼ cup plus 2 tablespoons unrefined coconut oil

2 tablespoons beeswax

50 drops eucalyptus essential oil

25 drops peppermint essential oil

15 drops lavender essential oil

15 drops sweet marjoram essential oil

Helpful Hint: To calm a cough at bedtime, massage the vapor rub into the bottoms of your feet and cover with socks.

Breathe Easy Shower Steamers

AROMATIC

Safe for ages 6+. Not safe for pregnant or nursing mothers

Showers are therapeutic for respiratory systems, especially in the case of cough and congestion. These shower steamers harness the power of steam and aromatherapy to help you breathe easier.

1. Wearing rubber or latex gloves, mix the baking soda, citric acid, and cornstarch in a medium-size bowl, breaking up any clumps with your fingers.

2. Add the essential oils to the mixture, and thoroughly stir them into the powders, breaking up small clumps with your gloved hands.

3. Using the bottle of witch hazel, spray the mixture 2 to 3 times and continue to mix using your gloved hands until it packs together (like a snowball) without crumbling.

4. Repeat step 3 if the mixture is too dry to hold together.

5. Pack the mixture into a ¼-cup measuring cup, making sure to press it in firmly. Gently turn out onto parchment paper or wax paper to dry. If using silicone molds, pack the mixture firmly into the molds, and let dry overnight before popping them out.

6. Place one shower steamer at the end of the bathtub or shower, avoiding direct contact with the water. Let it slowly dissolve while you shower, and breathe in the aroma.

Makes 6 to 8 shower steamers

1 cup baking soda

½ cup citric acid

1 tablespoon cornstarch (can be substituted with arrowroot powder or any type of clay)

½ teaspoon eucalyptus essential oil

½ teaspoon lavender essential oil

Witch hazel in a small spray bottle

¼-cup measuring cup or silicone molds

Helpful Hint: While stored, the scent will eventually evaporate. If this happens, simply add a few drops of each essential oil to the top of the shower steamer before using.

Cooling Fever Compress

TOPICAL

Safe for ages 6+. Not safe for pregnant or nursing mothers

Fevers are your body's natural strategy for fighting infections, and, for the most part, they should be supported rather than reduced. A cooling compress can help bring down your body's temperature when it rises too high.

1. Mix the boiling water with the peppermint tea bag. Cover and steep for 15 to 20 minutes.

2. Add 1 to 2 cups of ice cubes, and stir until the ice is melted and the water temperature is cool but not ice cold.

3. Mix the essential oils and apple cider vinegar into the cool peppermint tea, and stir to blend.

4. Dip a washcloth into the mixture and squeeze out excess water. Apply to the forehead and feet to help draw heat from the body.

Makes 1 treatment

2 cups boiling water

1 peppermint tea bag (or
   1 tablespoon loose leaf tea)

1 to 2 cups ice cubes

4 drops peppermint
   essential oil

4 drops lavender essential oil

¼ cup raw apple cider vinegar

Substitution Tip: For a kid-friendly cooling fever compress, substitute spearmint essential oil for the peppermint essential oil.

Soothing Cold and Flu Bath

TOPICAL

Safe for ages 2+

Baths are my first line of defense whenever someone in my family has a cold or flu. This soothing blend helps alleviate cold and flu symptoms while relaxing the body and supporting the immune system.

Makes 1 treatment

2 tablespoons sweet almond oil (or another liquid carrier oil)

3 drops rosalina essential oil

3 drops sweet marjoram essential oil

3 drops lavender essential oil

1 cup Epsom salt

1. In a medium-size bowl, stir together the carrier oil and essential oils.

2. Using a spoon, stir Epsom salt into the oil mixture.

3. Pour the mixture under running bath water.

4. Soak in the tub for at least 20 minutes.

Substitution Tip: If you don't want a slippery tub after the bath, substitute your favorite unscented shampoo or bubble bath for the carrier oil in this recipe.

Earache Oil

Makes 1 ounce

Safe for ages 2+. Check with your doctor before use to be sure the eardrum is not perforated. Not for use with ear tubes

Earaches and infections are no fun for anyone, no matter their age. This oil is designed to relieve the pain of earaches and treat ear infections with antibacterial and antiviral essential oils diluted at 2 percent in olive oil.

1. Add the olive oil and essential oils to a 1-ounce glass bottle with a dropper lid.

2. Gently swirl to blend.

3. Warm the oil first by sealing it in a plastic bag and submerging it in a bowl of warm water. Gently tilt the head to the side, and put 1 or 2 drops into the ear. Keep the head tilted for two minutes before repeating with the other ear. This can be used twice a day, as needed.

2 tablespoons extra virgin olive oil

6 drops lavender essential oil

6 drops rosalina essential oil

3 drops tea tree essential oil

3 drops Roman chamomile essential oil

Helpful Hint: You also can massage 1 to 3 drops of oil around the outside of the ear and down the neck, as needed.

Antibacterial "Owie" Salve

TOPICAL

Safe for all ages

This all-purpose healing salve soothes and treats skin abrasions, cuts, and other types of "owies."

1. In a pan over low heat, melt the coconut oil, shea butter, and beeswax.

2. Once melted, remove from heat, and add the essential oils. Stir until thoroughly blended.

3. Pour into a 4-ounce mason jar, and put into the freezer for about 20 minutes to harden.

4. To use, apply a small, pea-size amount to clean wounds, cuts, scrapes, and other types of "owies."

Makes about 4 ounces

¼ cup unrefined coconut oil
2 tablespoons shea butter
2 tablespoons beeswax
30 drops lavender essential oil
30 drops tea tree essential oil
20 drops lemon essential oil

Helpful Hint: Pour the salve mixture into ½-ounce metal tins or empty lip balm tubes for an on-the-go version that you can keep in your purse or backpack.

Antibacterial Cleansing Wound Spray

TOPICAL

Safe for all ages

The first step to healing a wound without infection is cleaning it properly. With this antibacterial spray, you can quickly clean any wound, whether you're at home or out in the wilderness.

1. In a 4-ounce spray bottle, mix the witch hazel, aloe vera gel, and vegetable glycerin with the essential oils. Gently swirl to blend.

2. Add enough distilled water to fill the bottle.

3. Shake well and spray onto open or dirty wounds. Gently pat dry with a clean cloth or towel. Follow with Antibacterial "Owie" Salve. Store any unused spray in a cool, dark location.

Makes 4 ounces

¼ cup witch hazel
1 tablespoon aloe vera gel
1 teaspoon vegetable glycerin
6 drops geranium essential oil
10 drops lavender essential oil
10 drops rosalina essential oil
Distilled water, to fill

Substitution Tip: For extra healing benefits, substitute lavender or calendula hydrosol for distilled water. Both are known to help boost tissue regeneration, soothe inflammation, and treat wounds.

Anti-Itch Calamine Lotion

Clay and herbs traditionally have been used to soothe itching, and the remedy today is not much different. This lotion is used around the world to soothe itchy bug bites, rashes, poison ivy/oak, and chicken pox.

1. In a small glass bowl, mix the baking soda and bentonite clay, then stir in the vegetable glycerin.

2. Slowly (1 tablespoon at a time) add the witch hazel, and stir until a smooth and creamy paste forms.

3. Add the coconut oil and essential oils, and stir them into the paste.

4. Apply to itchy bug bites, rashes, chicken pox, and more. Refrigerate when not in use.

Makes about 4 ounces

2 tablespoons baking soda

3 tablespoons bentonite clay

1 tablespoon vegetable glycerin

Enough witch hazel to form a paste

1 teaspoon unrefined coconut oil, melted but not hot

15 drops lavender essential oil

5 drops tea tree essential oil

Seasonal Allergies Personal Inhaler

AROMATIC

Safe for ages 6+. Not safe for pregnant or
nursing mothers

*Seasonal allergies bring itchy noses, sniffles, and watery
eyes, but a personal aromatherapy inhaler can help discreetly soothe those symptoms, no matter where you are.
Small and compact, it can be carried in your pocket, purse,
briefcase, or backpack.*

1. Mix all the essential oils in a small glass bowl.
2. Using tweezers, add the wick (the cotton pad) of an aromatherapy personal inhaler to the bowl, and roll it around until the essential oil mixture is absorbed.
3. Use the tweezers to transfer the wick to the inhaler tube. Close the tube, and label the inhaler.
4. Take a whiff of the inhaler as needed.

Makes 1 treatment

5 drops eucalyptus
    essential oil
5 drops lemon essential oil
5 drops rosalina essential oil
5 drops cypress essential oil
1 clean wick for personal
    aromatherapy inhaler

Substitution Tip: For a kid-
and pregnancy-friendly
version, substitute blue
tansy essential oil for the
eucalyptus essential oil.
Though most companies only
sell blue tansy (*Tanacetum
annuum*), be careful not
to confuse this with tansy
(*Tanacetum vulgare*) oil.

Headache and Sinus Roll-On

TOPICAL

Safe for ages 6+. Not safe for pregnant or
nursing mothers

*Headaches and migraines are the worst, and this is my
go-to blend. Peppermint essential oil is well known for its
ability to soothe a headache, while lavender helps to relax
tension, and eucalyptus eases sinus pressure.*

1. Add the essential oils to a ⅓-ounce glass
   roll-on bottle.

2. Add enough fractionated coconut oil to fill the
   bottle. Attach the roller ball and cap, and gently
   swirl to blend. Don't forget to label the bottle.

3. Roll onto your temples and the back of your neck.
   Gently massage.

Makes ⅓ ounce

3 drops peppermint
   essential oil
3 drops lavender essential oil
3 drops eucalyptus
   essential oil
Fractionated coconut oil, to fill

Muscle Mender Bath

TOPICAL

Safe for ages 2+

*After a hard day at work or tough workout at the gym, your
muscles could use some special attention, and an aromatherapeutic Epsom bath is exactly what they need. For
children between the ages of 2 and 6 years, subtract 1 drop
from each essential oil in the recipe.*

1. In a medium-size glass bowl, stir together the bubble
   bath and essential oils.

2. Using a spoon, stir the Epsom salt into the mixture.

3. Pour the mixture under running bath water.

4. Soak in the tub for at least 20 minutes.

Makes 1 treatment

2 tablespoons unscented
   bubble bath
3 drops sweet marjoram
   essential oil
3 drops rosalina essential oil
3 drops black pepper
   essential oil
1 cup Epsom salt

Helpful Hint: Substitute your
favorite carrier oil for the
bubble bath in this recipe,
if needed.

Muscle Mender Warming Massage Oil

TOPICAL

Safe for ages 6+. Not safe for pregnant or nursing mothers

When muscles ache, there's no better therapy than a massage. This oil will help warm the massage area, increase circulation, and reduce pain. For kid-friendly recipes, see chapter 7 for Growing Pains Bath (page 109) and Growing Pains Massage Oil (page 110).

1. In a medium glass bowl, stir together the carrier oil and essential oils.

2. Pour the mixture into a lotion pump bottle (or preferred container).

3. Massage the oil into achy muscles. Avoid getting it on any sensitive areas to prevent irritation. Store in a cool, dark location.

Makes about 2 ounces

¼ cup carrier oil

25 drops peppermint essential oil

20 drops clove bud essential oil

20 drops cinnamon leaf essential oil

15 drops ginger essential oil

Soothing Sore Throat Gargle

TOPICAL

Safe for ages 10+. Not safe for pregnant or nursing mothers

A sore throat is a real pain, but essential oils can help. Peppermint essential oil is helpful for soothing a sore throat because it reduces inflammation and cools the pain while also boosting the immune system to help fight off infection.

1. Dilute the peppermint essential oil in the fractionated coconut oil. Pour the mixture into a bottle.

2. Gargle the oil for 30 seconds, then spit. Do not swallow the mixture. Store in a cool, dark location.

Makes 1 ounce

9 drops peppermint essential oil

2 tablespoons fractionated coconut oil

Substitution Tip: Substitute spearmint or lemon essential oil if peppermint is too strong for your taste buds.

Antifungal Salve

Makes about 4 ounces

Safe for ages 2+

With persistence and highly antifungal essential oils, you can get rid of athlete's foot, ringworm, and other types of skin fungi that are difficult to treat. This salve soothes inflamed skin while combating fungal infections and relieving itching.

1. In a pan over low heat, melt the coconut oil, shea butter, and beeswax.

2. Once melted, remove from heat, add the essential oils, and stir.

3. Pour into a 4-ounce mason jar, and put into the freezer for about 20 minutes to harden.

4. Apply a pea-size amount to clean and dry skin twice a day.

¼ cup unrefined coconut oil

2 tablespoons shea butter

2 tablespoons beeswax

30 drops lavender essential oil

30 drops tea tree essential oil

20 drops cinnamon leaf essential oil

Helpful Hint: Pour the salve mixture into ½-ounce metal tins or empty lip balm tubes to use on the go.

Wart Remover Oil

TOPICAL

Makes ⅓ ounce

Safe for ages 2+. Do not apply to genitals

Warts can be extremely difficult to get rid of, but I've seen essential oils magically dissolve them without any painful procedures. This oil also helps with skin tags.

1. Add the essential oils to an empty ⅓-ounce glass bottle with a dropper.

2. Add enough fractionated coconut oil to fill the bottle. Insert the dropper cap, and gently swirl to blend. Don't forget a label.

3. Apply a couple of drops to a cotton ball, and place it on the wart two to three times daily until it disappears.

30 drops lemon essential oil (steam-distilled)

25 drops cypress essential oil

25 drops sweet marjoram essential oil

15 drops tea tree essential oil

Fractionated coconut oil, to fill

Eczema Balm

Makes about ¼ ounce

When you have an eczema flare-up, this soothing balm helps reduce inflammation, stop itching, and heal blisters.

¼ cup unrefined coconut oil

2 tablespoons shea butter

2 tablespoons beeswax

40 drops lavender essential oil

25 drops geranium essential oil

25 drops coriander essential oil

10 drops Atlas cedarwood essential oil

1. In a pan over low heat, melt the coconut oil, shea butter, and beeswax.
2. Once melted, remove from heat, and add the essential oils. Stir to blend.
3. Pour into a 4-ounce mason jar, and put into the freezer for about 20 minutes to harden.
4. Apply a pea-size amount to affected areas, as needed.

Anti-Nausea Personal Inhaler

Makes 1 treatment

Nausea can strike at any moment, and it helps to have the appropriate essential oils on hand. Mint and ginger are well known for their digestive capabilities, and together they calm the worst of nausea, including seasickness and motion sickness. You can carry this personal inhaler in your purse, briefcase, backpack, or pocket for discreet and easy access.

10 drops peppermint essential oil

7 drops spearmint essential oil

3 drops ginger essential oil

1 clean wick for personal aromatherapy inhaler

1. Mix the essential oils in a small glass bowl.
2. Using tweezers, add the wick (the cotton pad) of an aromatherapy personal inhaler to the bowl, and roll it around until the essential oil mixture is absorbed.
3. Use the tweezers to transfer the wick to the inhaler tube. Close the tube, and label the inhaler.
4. Inhale, as needed.

Tummy Tamer Roll-On

TOPICAL

Safe for ages 2+. Not safe for pregnant or
nursing mothers

*In the case of an upset stomach, indigestion, or gas,
apply this roll-on to the abdomen to help calm a queasy
stomach. It also can double as a personal inhaler to quickly
soothe nausea.*

1. Add the essential oils to a ⅓-ounce glass
   roll-on bottle.

2. Add enough fractionated coconut oil to fill the
   bottle. Attach the roller ball and cap, and gently
   swirl to blend. Don't forget to add a label.

3. Roll onto your abdomen, and gently massage clock-
   wise in a circular motion.

Makes ⅓ ounce

5 drops spearmint essential oil

5 drops sweet orange
    essential oil

3 drops ginger essential oil

2 drops lemongrass
    essential oil

Fractionated coconut oil, to fill

CHAPTER SIX:

For Emotional Well-Being

Stress/Anxiety Diffuser Blend

AROMATIC

Safe for all ages. Not safe for pregnant mothers

When stress and anxiety run high, this diffuser blend can help release tension, calm hormonal mood swings, and soothe frazzled nerves.

1. Add all the essential oils to an empty essential oil bottle (or any dark glass bottle with a dropper), and gently swirl the bottle to blend.

2. Add 8 to 10 drops to a diffuser, and diffuse in 30-minute increments (30 minutes on/30 minutes off).

Makes ½ ounce

1 teaspoon lavender essential oil

½ teaspoon clary sage essential oil

1 teaspoon grapefruit essential oil

½ teaspoon Roman chamomile essential oil

Helpful Hint: This essential oil blend can be used in an aromatherapy roll-on, too. Add 9 drops of the blend to a ⅓-ounce glass roll-on bottle and fill with fractionated coconut oil.

Antianxiety Shower Steamers

AROMATIC

Safe for all ages

There's nothing better than relaxing with a shower steamer. These steamers are bright and citrusy and great for relieving stress and anxiety. Sit back in the shower, and let aromatherapy wash away your worries.

1. Wearing rubber or latex gloves, mix baking soda, citric acid, and cornstarch in a medium-size bowl, breaking up any clumps with your fingers.

2. Add the essential oils to the mixture, and thoroughly mix them into the powders, breaking up small clumps.

3. Using the bottle of witch hazel, spray the mixture 2 to 3 times and continue to mix using your gloved hands until it packs together (like a snowball) without crumbling.

4. Repeat step 3 if the mixture is too dry to hold together.

5. Pack ¼ cup of the mixture into a measuring cup, making sure to press the mixture firmly, and gently turn out onto parchment paper or wax paper to dry. If using silicone molds, pack the mixture firmly into the molds, and let dry overnight before popping them out.

6. Place one shower steamer at the end of the bathtub or shower, avoiding direct contact with the water. Let it slowly dissolve while you shower, and deeply inhale the aroma.

Makes 6 to 8 shower steamers

1 cup baking soda

½ cup citric acid

1 tablespoon cornstarch (can be substituted with arrowroot powder or any type of clay)

½ teaspoon bergamot essential oil

½ teaspoon coriander essential oil

Witch hazel in a small spray bottle

¼-cup measuring cup or silicone molds

Relaxer Roll-On

TOPICAL

Safe for ages 2+

Use the relaxer roll-on, with its calming floral and citrus aromas, to calm your nerves and soothe your worries.

1. Add the essential oils to a ⅓-ounce glass roll-on bottle.

2. Add enough fractionated coconut oil to fill the bottle. Attach the roller ball and cap, and gently swirl to blend. Don't forget to add a label.

3. Roll and gently massage the oil onto your temples, wrists, and the back of your neck.

Makes ⅓ ounce

3 drops Roman chamomile essential oil

3 drops sweet orange essential oil

3 drops geranium essential oil

Fractionated coconut oil, to fill

Happy Day Roll-On Perfume

TOPICAL

Safe for ages 6+. Not safe for pregnant or nursing mothers

Start your day off on the right side of the bed with a fresh and uplifting perfume that will delight your senses.

1. Add the essential oils to a ⅓-ounce glass roll-on bottle.

2. Add enough grapeseed oil to fill the bottle. Attach the roller ball and cap, and gently swirl to blend. Don't forget to add a label.

3. Apply it like a perfume: behind ears and on wrists, cleavage, and the nape of the neck. Natural perfumes don't last as long as synthetic perfumes, so reapply as often as needed.

Makes ⅓ ounce

3 drops grapefruit essential oil

2 drops coriander essential oil

3 drops bergamot essential oil

1 drop lemongrass essential oil

Grapeseed oil, to fill

Substitution Tip: Grapeseed oil is used in this recipe to carry the scent longer, but feel free to use another liquid carrier oil, such as fractionated coconut oil.

Sunshine and Rainbows Body Spray

Safe for ages 2+

When you're feeling blue, this sweet-smelling blend will lift your spirits.

1. In a 4-ounce spray bottle, mix the witch hazel, aloe vera gel, and vegetable glycerin with the essential oils. Gently swirl to blend.

2. Add enough distilled water to fill the bottle.

3. Shake well before spraying onto your clothing or body. Store in a cool, dark location.

Makes 4 ounces

¼ cup witch hazel

1 tablespoon aloe vera gel

1 teaspoon vegetable glycerin

40 drops lemon essential oil

50 drops bergamot
   essential oil

2 drops ylang-ylang
   essential oil

15 drops vanilla essential oil

Distilled water, to fill

Helpful Hint: You can use this spray on pillows, couches, towels, and bedding.

Magnesium Bedtime Spray

TOPICAL

Safe for ages 2+

Magnesium deficiency is extremely common and can cause various symptoms including migraines, anxiety, mood swings, insomnia, and muscle spasms. This bedtime spray combines the power of relaxing essential oils and magnesium to help calm and soothe your mind and body for sleep.

1. In a 4-ounce spray bottle, mix the jojoba oil and vegetable glycerin with the essential oils. Gently swirl to blend.

2. Add enough magnesium oil to fill the bottle.

3. Apply at bedtime. Shake well, and spray onto your entire body, especially your arms, legs, and feet. Massage into your skin. Store in a cool, dark location.

Makes 4 ounces

1 tablespoon jojoba oil

1 teaspoon vegetable glycerin

40 drops lavender essential oil

20 drops sweet marjoram essential oil

15 drops Atlas cedarwood essential oil

30 drops sweet orange essential oil

Magnesium oil, to fill

Note: If you are new to using a magnesium spray, your skin may begin to itch. If that occurs, dilute the recipe in your first bottle with 2 tablespoons of distilled water before filling it with the magnesium oil. You can use the recipe at regular strength when it's time to refill your bottle.

Helpful Hint: You can use store-bought magnesium oil or easily make it yourself. To make your own magnesium oil, mix ½ magnesium flakes (magnesium chloride, not Epsom salt) with 3 tablespoons of boiling water, and stir until completely dissolved.

Sleep Deep Bedtime Bath

TOPICAL

Safe for ages 2+

A bath can help you unwind, and this recipe is how I wash away a restless mind and stress before bedtime.

1. In a medium-size bowl, stir together the bubble bath and essential oils.
2. Using a spoon, stir Epsom salt into the mixture.
3. Pour the blend under running bath water.
4. Soak for at least 20 minutes.

Makes 1 treatment

2 tablespoons unscented bubble bath or shampoo

3 drops lavender essential oil

3 drops Roman chamomile essential oil

3 drops coriander essential oil

1 cup Epsom salt

Helpful Hint: If you don't have any bubble bath on hand, feel free to substitute your favorite carrier oil.

Calming Bedtime Pillow Spray

AROMATIC

Safe for ages 2+

Setting the right atmosphere for sleep is one of the first steps to getting a better night's rest. This remedy can be sprayed all around your bedroom to create a calming atmosphere. I add rosalina essential oil to relieve congestion and reduce snoring, as needed.

1. In a 4-ounce spray bottle, mix the witch hazel with the essential oils. Gently swirl to blend.
2. Add enough distilled water to fill the bottle.
3. Shake well, and spray onto bedding (pillows, blankets, sheets, mattress, bedroom curtains). Store in a cool, dark location.

Makes 4 ounces

¼ cup witch hazel

40 drops lavender essential oil

40 drops bergamot essential oil

20 drops Roman chamomile essential oil

10 drops rosalina essential oil

Distilled water, to fill

Helpful Hint: Before bedtime, spray this oil blend on your pajamas and toss them into the dryer for five minutes. It will warm them and provide a lovely soothing scent to help lull you to sleep.

Sleepytime Massage Oil

TOPICAL

Safe for ages 2+

Many of us carry stress in our muscles. A massage with this oil and its fresh, woody aroma before bedtime can help relieve tension, allowing you to fall asleep faster.

1. In a medium glass bowl, stir together the carrier oil and essential oils.

2. Pour the mixture into a lotion pump bottle (or preferred container).

3. Massage the oil into your body, focusing on the shoulders, neck, legs, and feet. Avoid any sensitive areas. Store in a cool, dark location.

Makes about 2 ounces

¼ cup carrier oil

15 drops lavender essential oil

10 drops sweet marjoram essential oil

10 drops Atlas cedarwood essential oil

5 drops frankincense essential oil

Morning Time Yoga Mat Spray

AROMATIC, TOPICAL, CLEANING

Safe for ages 2+, Not safe for pregnant or nursing mothers

Yoga is the perfect way to start the day. This fresh, energizing yoga mat spray is multi-purpose and can be used to set the mood before your practice and to clean your mat afterward.

1. In a 4-ounce spray bottle, mix the witch hazel with the essential oils. Gently swirl to blend.

2. Add enough distilled water to fill the bottle.

3. Shake well, and spray the mat and yourself before beginning your yoga practice. Afterward, spray the mat thoroughly, and pat it dry with a towel.

Makes 4 ounces

¼ cup witch hazel

20 drops grapefruit essential oil

20 drops lemon essential oil

10 drops spearmint essential oil

5 drops basil essential oil

Distilled water, to fill

Mindful Meditation Roll-On

Safe for ages 2+. Not safe for pregnant mothers

This aromatherapy roll-on will help you reap the deep benefits of meditation by grounding you and helping increase focus and concentration.

1. Add the essential oils to a ⅓-ounce glass roll-on bottle.

2. Add enough fractionated coconut oil to fill the bottle. Attach the roller ball and cap, and gently swirl to blend. Don't forget to add a label.

3. As you prepare to meditate, gently massage the oil onto your temples, forehead, neck, and the bottoms of your feet.

Makes ⅓ ounce

1 drop frankincense
  essential oil
3 drops bergamot essential oil
3 drops lavender essential oil
2 drops clary sage
  essential oil
Fractionated coconut oil, to fill

Energy-Boosting Shower Steamers

AROMATIC

Safe for ages 6+. Not safe for pregnant mothers

Every morning, I take coffee or tea with me into the shower after tossing in one of these energy-boosting shower steamers. Then, I apply hair conditioner and sit sipping my drink and inhaling the energizing aromas of peppermint, lemon, and rosemary. It's a blissful way to start the day!

1. Wearing rubber or latex gloves, mix together baking soda, citric acid, and cornstarch in a medium-size bowl, breaking up any clumps with your fingers.

2. Add the essential oils to the blend and thoroughly stir them into the powders, breaking up small clumps.

3. Using the bottle of witch hazel, spray the mixture 2 to 3 times and continue to mix using your gloved hands until it will pack together (like a snowball) without crumbling.

4. Repeat step 3 if the mixture still is too dry to hold together.

5. Pack ¼ cup of the mixture into a measuring cup, making sure to press it firmly, and gently turn out onto parchment paper or wax paper to dry. If using silicone molds, pack the mixture firmly into the molds, and let dry overnight before popping them out.

6. Place a shower steamer at the end of the bathtub or shower, avoiding direct contact with the water. Let it slowly dissolve while you shower and inhale the aroma.

Makes 6 to 8 shower steamers

1 cup baking soda

½ cup citric acid

1 tablespoon cornstarch (can be substituted with arrowroot powder or any type of clay)

½ teaspoon lemon essential oil

¼ teaspoon peppermint essential oil

¼ teaspoon rosemary essential oil

Witch hazel in a small spray bottle

¼-cup measuring cup or silicone molds

Go Go Go Personal Inhaler

AROMATIC

Safe for ages 6+. Not safe for pregnant mothers

We've all experienced that midday slump when we'd rather be napping than at work or school. This blend is designed to get you through times when you need to add a little pep to your step.

1. Mix all the essential oils in a small glass bowl.
2. Using tweezers, add the wick (the cotton pad) of an aromatherapy personal inhaler to the bowl, and roll it around until the essential oil mixture is absorbed.
3. Use the tweezers to transfer the wick to the inhaler tube. Close the tube, and label the inhaler.
4. Inhale, as needed.

Makes 1 treatment

5 drops peppermint essential oil

5 drops fir needle essential oil

5 drops cypress essential oil

5 drops black pepper essential oil

1 clean wick for personal aromatherapy inhaler

Attention and Focus Roll-On

TOPICAL

Safe for ages 6+. Not safe for pregnant or nursing mothers

We all need a little help focusing every once in a while, and research shows certain essential oils—particularly cedarwood—can help increase cognitive function, clear brain fog, and reduce symptoms of ADHD.

1. Add the essential oils to a ⅓-ounce glass roll-on bottle.
2. Add fractionated coconut oil to fill the bottle. Attach the roller ball and cap, and gently swirl to blend. Don't forget to add a label.
3. Use the roll-on to gently massage oil onto your temples and the back of your neck.

Makes ⅓ ounce

3 drops Atlas cedarwood essential oil

3 drops bergamot essential oil

2 drops coriander essential oil

1 drop basil essential oil

Fractionated coconut oil, to fill

Homework Helper Diffuser Blend

AROMATIC

Safe for ages 2+

When it's crunch time at school and you have projects due, this diffuser blend can help you focus on the task at hand. Diffuse this blend at home or in the classroom to enhance concentration and increase productivity. This diffuser blend can also be used in the office to help keep you focused at work.

1. Add all the essential oils to an empty essential oil bottle (or any dark glass bottle with a dropper), and gently swirl to blend.

2. Add 8 to 10 drops to a diffuser, and diffuse in 30-minute increments (30 minutes on/ 30 minutes off).

Makes ½ ounce

1 teaspoon Atlas cedarwood essential oil

½ teaspoon lavender essential oil

½ teaspoon bergamot essential oil

½ teaspoon grapefruit essential oil

½ teaspoon frankincense essential oil

Helpful Hint: Try putting 25 drops of this blend in a personal inhaler for on-the-go relief.

Curb Your Appetite Personal Inhaler

AROMATIC

Safe for ages 2+

More than 90 percent of our sense of taste is smell-related, and pleasant aromas can send a signal to the brain that our appetite is appeased, even if we haven't taken a single bite of food. This recipe is designed to curb your appetite and put a halt to the munchies with repeated use.

1. Mix all the essential oils in a small glass bowl.

2. Using tweezers, add the wick (the cotton pad) of an aromatherapy personal inhaler to the bowl and roll it around until the essential oil mixture is absorbed.

3. Use the tweezers to transfer the wick to the inhaler tube. Close the tube, and label the inhaler.

4. Inhale, as needed.

Makes 1 treatment

5 drops grapefruit essential oil

5 drops bergamot essential oil

5 drops cinnamon leaf essential oil

5 drops coriander essential oil

1 clean wick for personal aromatherapy inhaler

Sweethearts' Dance Romance Massage Oil

TOPICAL

Safe for ages 2+

Makes 2 ounces

¼ cup carrier oil

25 drops bergamot essential oil

20 drops coriander essential oil

20 drops lavender essential oil

10 drops rose essential oil

You don't need a five-star hotel or fancy spa to enjoy a sensual experience. You easily can create a romantic atmosphere at home using essential oils. Toss some rose petals on the bed, light candles, and turn up your favorite music because this massage oil will light a spark.

1. In a medium glass bowl, stir together the carrier oil and essential oils.

2. Pour the mixture into a lotion pump bottle (or preferred container).

3. Massage the oil onto your partner's body, avoiding sensitive areas. Store in a cool, dark location.

Substitution Tip: Rose essential oil can be quite expensive, even for a small amount. Rose absolute is a fine substitution and smells just as heavenly.

Paradise Cove Romantic Room Spray

AROMATIC

Safe for ages 2+

Makes 4 ounces

¼ cup witch hazel

75 drops sweet orange essential oil

25 drops vanilla essential oil

10 drops ylang-ylang essential oil

Distilled water, to fill

Bring on the romance with this fragrant spray that can be applied to furniture, clothing, and bedding.

1. In a 4-ounce spray bottle, mix the witch hazel with the essential oils. Gently swirl to blend.

2. Add enough distilled water to fill the bottle.

3. Shake well, and spray in the air and on bedroom pillows, blankets, sheets, mattress, and curtains. Store in a cool, dark location.

Substitution Tip: Rose hydrosol pairs well with this spray and can be substituted for filtered water.

Spa Day Bath

TOPICAL

Safe for ages 6+. Not safe for pregnant or
nursing mothers

*When you need a spa day at home, this bath blend will do
the trick with soothing, uplifting aromas.*

1. In a medium-size bowl, stir together the carrier oil
   and essential oils.

2. Using a spoon, stir Epsom salt into the oil mixture.

3. Pour the mixture under running bath water.

4. Soak in the tub for at least 20 minutes.

Makes 1 treatment

2 tablespoons olive oil (or
  another liquid carrier oil)

3 drops lavender essential oil

3 drops eucalyptus
  essential oil

3 drops sweet marjoram
  essential oil

1 cup Epsom salt

Helpful Hint: Substitute
unscented shampoo or
bubble bath for the carrier oil
to avoid a slippery bathtub
after your soak.

Muse Creativity Perfume

TOPICAL

Safe for ages 6+. Not safe for pregnant or
nursing women

*This blend is an easy, effective, and natural method for
boosting inspiration and creativity, whether or not you're
an artist.*

1. Add the essential oils to a ⅓-ounce glass
   roll-on bottle.

2. Add grapeseed oil to fill the bottle. Attach the roller
   ball and cap, and gently swirl to blend. Don't forget
   to add a label.

3. Apply as you would a perfume: behind your ears, and
   on your wrists, cleavage, and the nape your neck.
   Natural perfumes do not last as long as synthetic
   perfumes, so reapply as often as needed.

Makes ⅓ ounce

3 drops sweet orange
  essential oil

2 drops bergamot essential oil

2 drops cinnamon leaf
  essential oil

1 drop clove bud essential oil

1 drop vanilla essential oil

Grapeseed oil, to fill

Substitution Tip: Grapeseed
oil helps maintain the scent
of this perfume, but another
liquid carrier oil, such as
fractionated coconut oil, may
be used.

CHAPTER SEVEN:

For the Family

Stretch Mark Balm

Safe for all ages

Stretch marks and scars are natural parts of pregnancy and childbirth, but they can be minimized with care. Daily application of this stretch mark balm can prevent and reduce fine lines, scars, and stretch marks, and it's safe for the whole family.

1. In a pan over low heat, melt the coconut oil and mango butter.

2. Once melted, remove from heat and stir in the rosehip seed oil, vitamin E, and essential oils.

3. Pour into a mason jar, and put into the freezer for about 20 minutes to harden.

4. Massage onto your belly, back, butt, arms, and legs daily to prevent stretch marks and reduce scarring.

Makes about 5 ounces

2 tablespoons unrefined coconut oil

¼ cup mango butter

¼ cup rosehip seed oil

1 teaspoon vitamin E

15 drops lavender essential oil

10 drops lemon essential oil

5 drops Roman chamomile essential oil

Substitution Tip: Tamanu oil has been studied extensively over the last 20 years, and evidence shows it has an amazing ability to treat damaged skin, including stretch marks and scars. Substitute 2 tablespoons of tamanu oil for half of the rosehip seed oil in this recipe to boost its healing benefits.

Morning Sickness Personal Inhaler

AROMATIC

Safe for all ages

More than half of all pregnant women experience morning sickness, and essential oil inhalers are a great way to help relieve symptoms. This personal inhaler recipe gives you a compact option that can discreetly be carried in a purse, briefcase, backpack, or pocket.

1. Mix all the essential oils in a small glass bowl.

2. Using tweezers, add the wick (the cotton pad) of an aromatherapy personal inhaler to the bowl and roll it around until the essential oil mixture is absorbed.

3. Use the tweezers to transfer the wick to the inhaler tube. Close the tube and label the inhaler.

4. Inhale, as needed.

Makes 1 treatment

10 drops coriander
   essential oil

10 drops ginger essential oil

10 drops lemon essential oil

1 clean wick for personal
   aromatherapy inhaler

Bohemi Mama's Boobie Balm

TOPICAL

Safe for all ages

Nursing your baby is a beautiful experience, but its down-sides include dry, cracked nipples and the occasional bite marks. This soothing boobie balm is designed to relieve and treat sore breasts and leave skin soft and supple.

1. In a pan over low heat, melt the coconut oil, shea butter, and beeswax.

2. Once melted, remove from heat, and add the essential oils. Stir to blend.

3. Pour into a 4-ounce mason jar, and put into the freezer for about 20 minutes to harden.

4. Apply a pea-size amount to breasts and nipples immediately after nursing and before the next feeding.

Makes 4 ounces

¼ cup unrefined coconut oil

2 tablespoons shea butter

2 tablespoons beeswax

16 drops lavender essential oil

20 drops Roman chamomile essential oil

Helpful Hint: Pour the balm mixture into ½-ounce metal tins or empty lip balm tubes for on-the-go convenience.

Baby Powder

TOPICAL

Safe for all ages

Baby powder keeps little bottoms dry in their diapers and prevents diaper rash. Unlike many off-the-shelf baby pow-ders, this recipe is talc-free and easy to prepare.

1. Mix arrowroot powder and white kaolin clay in a medium-size bowl.

2. Add essential oil and blend into the clay using rubber or latex gloved hands, breaking up any clumps.

3. Pour the desired amount of powder on your baby's clean, dry bottom to wick away and absorb moisture and soften skin. Store in a powder container.

Makes 1 cup

½ cup arrowroot powder

½ cup white kaolin clay

20 drops sweet orange essential oil

Helpful Hint: Turn this blend into an awesome herbal baby powder by adding 1 table-spoon each of finely ground lavender buds, chamomile flowers, and comfrey leaves.

Plague Killer Jr. Diffuser Blend

AROMATIC

Safe for all ages

Nothing kills germs like this kid-friendly antibacterial and antiviral essential oil blend. Diffuse it throughout your home to support the immune system and ease cold and flu symptoms.

1. Add all the essential oils to an empty essential oil bottle (or any dark glass bottle with a dropper), and gently swirl to blend.

2. Add 6 to 8 drops to a diffuser, and diffuse in 30-minute increments (30 minutes on/30 minutes off).

Makes ½ ounce

¾ teaspoon lavender essential oil

1 teaspoon rosalina essential oil

¼ teaspoon fir needle essential oil

¾ teaspoon sweet marjoram essential oil

¼ teaspoon frankincense essential oil

Helpful Hint: This essential oil blend also can be used in any of this book's cleaning recipes.

Kids' Vapor Rub

TOPICAL

Safe for ages 2+

Vapor rubs are great remedies for respiratory illness, but it's not advised to use eucalyptus or peppermint essential oils around young children. This recipe features kid-friendly essential oils to help relieve cough and congestion and make it easier for little ones to breathe (see the recipe on page 74 for older children and adults).

1. In a pan over low heat, melt the coconut oil and beeswax.

2. Once melted, remove from heat, and add the essential oils.

3. Pour into a 4-ounce mason jar, and put into the freezer for about 20 minutes to harden.

4. Apply to the chest, back, and neck, as needed.

Makes about 4 ounces

¼ cup plus 2 tablespoons unrefined coconut oil

2 tablespoons beeswax

20 drops lavender essential oil

20 drops fir needle essential oil

20 drops spearmint essential oil

20 drops sweet marjoram essential oil

Helpful Hint: To calm a cough at bedtime, massage vapor rub into the soles of the feet and cover with socks.

Baby Butt Balm

Safe for all ages

This gentle balm naturally soothes and treats raw skin while keeping the area clean. It also doubles as a kid-friendly "owie" cream for cuts, scrapes, and other minor injuries.

1. In a pan over low heat, melt the coconut oil, shea butter, and beeswax.

2. Once melted, remove from heat, and add the essential oils. Stir to blend.

3. Pour into a 4-ounce mason jar, and put into the freezer for about 20 minutes to harden.

4. Apply a pea-size amount to a clean and dry butt to soothe inflammation and prevent rashes.

Makes about 4 ounces

¼ cup unrefined coconut oil

2 tablespoons shea butter

2 tablespoons beeswax

12 drops lavender essential oil

12 drops Roman chamomile essential oil

Helpful Hint: Pour the balm mixture into ½-ounce metal tins or empty lip balm tubes to take on the road.

Teething Roll-On

TOPICAL

Safe for ages 6+ months. For external use only

Teething can be a tough time for babies and parents. While some recommend using clove bud essential oil to numb baby's gums, it's not a safe practice. Essential oils should be used only externally to soothe teething pain. This topical roll-on is applied on the jawline and cheeks to relieve pain and restore calm.

Makes ½ ounce

1 drop lavender essential oil

1 drop Roman chamomile essential oil

1 drop rosalina essential oil

Fractionated coconut oil, to fill

1. Add the essential oils to a ⅓-ounce glass roll-on bottle.

2. Add fractionated coconut oil to fill the bottle. Attach the roller ball and cap, and gently swirl to blend. Don't forget to add a label.

3. Gently roll onto the jawline/cheek area as often as needed.

Growing Pains Bath

TOPICAL

Safe for ages 2+

Although we refer to them as "growing pains," the cramping aches experienced by children ages 3 to 12 in their arms and legs seem to be more common after especially active days. This bath will help ease pain and relax muscles so that your child can get a better night's sleep.

1. In a medium-size bowl, stir together the bubble bath and essential oils.

2. Using a spoon, stir the Epsom salt into the mixture.

3. Pour the mixture under running bath water.

4. Soak in the tub for at least 20 minutes.

Makes 1 treatment

2 tablespoons unscented bubble bath

2 drops sweet marjoram essential oil

2 drops rosalina essential oil

2 drops lavender essential oil

1 cup Epsom salt

Helpful Hint:
Anti-inflammatory herbs such as lavender and chamomile make awesome additions to this bath. Add ¼ cup of each herb to a cloth tea bag or an old, clean sock tied closed before tossing into the bathtub.

Growing Pains Massage Oil

TOPICAL

Safe for ages 2+

Growing pains seem to strike in the evening, and this remedy will not only calm and soothe sore muscles but also relax a child before bedtime.

1. In a medium glass bowl, stir together the carrier oil and essential oils.

2. Pour the mixture into a lotion pump bottle (or preferred container).

3. Massage the oil into your child's achy muscles, avoiding sensitive areas. Store in a cool, dark location.

Makes 2 ounces

¼ cup carrier oil

10 drops lavender essential oil

15 drops sweet marjoram essential oil

10 drops Roman chamomile essential oil

Helpful Hint: For best results, use this massage oil after a Growing Pains Bath (see page 109).

Aunt Flo's Soothing Salve

Safe for ages 10+. Not safe for pregnant women

I've experienced painful periods since I was a teenager and never wanted to take a lot of pills. This soothing salve helps to naturally ease some of the pain of menstruation.

1. In a pan over low heat, combine the olive oil and beeswax.

2. Once melted, remove from heat, and add the essential oils.

3. Pour into a 4-ounce mason jar, and put into the freezer for about 20 minutes to harden.

4. Apply to your abdomen, lower back, and thighs to reduce painful cramping and soothe frazzled nerves.

Makes about 4 ounces

¼ cup plus 2 tablespoons olive oil

2 tablespoons beeswax

30 drops clove bud essential oil

20 drops lavender essential oil

15 drops geranium essential oil

15 drops bergamot essential oil

10 drops clary sage essential oil

10 drops ginger essential oil

Helpful Hint:
Arnica and St. John's Wort are herbs well known for their anti-inflammatory and pain-relieving properties. For a wonderful addition, steep 2 tablespoons of arnica flowers and 2 tablespoons of St. John's Wort in the olive oil over low heat for 2 hours. Strain, and continue with the recipe.

PMS Bath

TOPICAL

Safe for ages 2+. Not safe for pregnant women

I know from firsthand experience that this PMS bath provides emotional and physical relief, balances hormones, and eases aches and pains.

1. In a medium-size bowl, stir the bubble bath and essential oils to blend.
2. Using a spoon, stir the Epsom salt into the mixture.
3. Pour the mixture under running bath water.
4. Soak in the tub for at least 20 minutes.

Makes 1 treatment

2 tablespoons unscented bubble bath

3 drops lavender essential oil

3 drops Roman chamomile essential oil

3 drops clary sage essential oil

1 cup Epsom salt

Substitution Tip: Don't have bubble bath on hand? Substitute your favorite carrier oil for the bubble bath in this recipe.

Helpful Hint: Follow this bath with Aunt Flo's Soothing Salve (see page 111) for longer-lasting PMS relief.

Menopause Mood Booster Roll-On

TOPICAL

Safe for ages 6+. Not safe for pregnant women

While menopause symptoms can vary from woman to woman, mood swings often accompany hormonal shifts. This calming roll-on will help soothe frazzled nerves, ease grumpiness, and regulate hormonal secretions.

1. Add the essential oils to a ⅓-ounce glass roll-on bottle.

2. Add enough fractionated coconut oil to fill the bottle. Attach the roller ball and cap, and gently swirl to blend. Don't forget to add a label.

3. Gently massage into your temples, neck, and cleavage, and behind your ears.

Makes ⅓ ounce

3 drops lavender essential oil

3 drops clary sage
   essential oil

3 drops geranium essential oil

Fractionated coconut oil, to fill

Cool Your Flashes Cooling Spray

Safe for ages 6+. Not safe for pregnant women

This miraculous hot flash spray will help you cool off in an instant, no matter where you are.

1. In a 4-ounce spray bottle, mix the witch hazel, aloe vera gel, and vegetable glycerin with the essential oils. Gently swirl to mix.

2. Add enough distilled water to fill the bottle.

3. Shake well, and spray face, arms, chest, and the back of your neck as needed for hot flash relief. Make sure to keep your eyes closed when misting your face.

Makes 4 ounces

¼ cup witch hazel

1 tablespoon aloe vera gel

1 teaspoon vegetable glycerin

10 drops peppermint essential oil

10 drops lavender essential oil

10 drops clary sage essential oil

Distilled water, to fill

Substitution Tip: Peppermint hydrosol is very gentle and has a wonderful cooling effect that can be used topically to cool you off. Substitute peppermint hydrosol for the water in this recipe for a cooler effect.

Helpful Hint: Try storing this spray in the refrigerator for an even colder, more refreshing application.

Jock Itch Salve

Safe for ages 6+. Not safe for pregnant or nursing women

Jock itch, a type of ringworm, is caused by a fungus that thrives in warm, moist areas of the body. The highly antifungal and anti-inflammatory essential oils used in this salve are gentle enough to be applied to the groin area and will soothe and treat fungal infections. It can be used on other types of ringworm as well as athlete's foot.

1. In a pan over low heat, melt the coconut oil, shea butter, and beeswax.

2. Once melted, remove from heat, and add the essential oils. Stir to blend.

3. Pour into a 4-ounce mason jar, and put into the freezer for about 20 minutes to harden.

4. Apply a pea-size amount to clean, dry rashes and itchy skin.

Makes about 4 ounces

¼ cup unrefined coconut oil

2 tablespoons shea butter

2 tablespoons beeswax

10 drops lavender essential oil

10 drops tea tree essential oil

10 drops lemon essential oil

10 drops eucalyptus essential oil

Helpful Hint: Pour the salve mixture into ½-ounce metal tins or empty lip balm tubes for on-the-go convenience.

Tropic Thunder Beard Oil

TOPICAL

Safe for ages 6+. Not safe for pregnant or
nursing women

*Beard oil like this one helps to condition, smooth, and
straighten beards so that they don't look scraggly. It also
helps to moisturize and soothe skin underneath the beard,
preventing itchiness.*

1. In a medium glass bowl, stir together the carrier oils
   and essential oils.

2. Pour the mixture into a glass bottle with a dropper
   top, and label the bottle.

3. After dampening your beard, pour 5 to 8 drops
   (depending on beard size) into the palm of your
   hand and massage into the beard. Comb through
   completely with your fingers.

Makes 1 ounce

1 tablespoon hemp seed oil

½ tablespoon avocado oil

½ tablespoon apricot
   kernel oil

10 drops cypress essential oil

10 drop bergamot essential oil

3 drops clove bud essential oil

Substitution Tip: For
a refreshing woodsy aroma,
substitute 10 drops of fir
needle, 10 drops of cedarwood, and 3 drops of
peppermint essential oils
for the essential oils in the
original recipe.

Divine Elevation ED Diffuser Blend

Erectile dysfunction affects about 30 million men nation-wide, and it can happen at any age. Limited research suggests some essentials oils—including a combination of pumpkin and lavender oils—may reduce anxiety and increase penile blood flow (Hirsch, 2014). With that in mind, this diffuser blend was created to relieve stress and help you get in the mood.

Makes ½ ounce

1 teaspoon sweet orange essential oil

¾ teaspoon lavender essential oil

¾ teaspoon cinnamon leaf essential oil

¼ teaspoon clove bud essential oil

¼ teaspoon vanilla essential oil

1. Add all the essential oils to an empty essential oil bottle (or any dark glass bottle with a dropper), and gently swirl to blend.

2. Add 8 to 10 drops to a diffuser, and diffuse for 30 minutes in the room where it's needed.

Helpful Hint: This essential oil blend also can be used in a massage oil. Mix 1 ounce of your favorite carrier oil with 18 drops of this blend, and massage into the back, chest, legs, and feet prior to intercourse. Avoid sensitive areas, and do not apply to your private parts.

Aftershave Spray

TOPICAL

Safe for ages 6+. Not safe for pregnant or
nursing mothers

*Aftershave helps clean and soothe skin, treat cuts, and
close pores. This spray can help reduce razor burn, bumps,
and inflamed skin, too.*

1. In a 4-ounce spray bottle, mix the witch hazel, aloe
   vera gel, and vegetable glycerin with the essential
   oils. Gently swirl to blend.

2. Add enough distilled water to fill the bottle.

3. Shake well, and carefully spray onto the face with
   eyes closed. Gently pat dry with a clean cloth or
   towel. Store in a cool, dark location.

Makes 4 ounces

¼ cup witch hazel

1 tablespoon aloe vera gel

1 teaspoon vegetable glycerin

10 drops tea tree essential oil

10 drops peppermint
   essential oil

Distilled water, to fill

Substitution Tip: For an
extra soothing twist on this
aftershave, substitute peppermint hydrosol for the water
in this recipe. Peppermint is
naturally anti-inflammatory
and antibacterial and will help
clean and soothe any cuts.

Helpful Hint: See chapter 8 to
follow this spray with a moisturizing facial oil (page 131).

Arthritis Alleviation Salve

TOPICAL

Safe for ages 6+. Not safe for pregnant or
nursing mothers

*Arthritis and joint pain can impede the simplest of tasks,
but certain essential oils—including lavender, ginger, and
frankincense—are very effective at soothing pain, reducing
inflammation, and helping you get through everyday tasks.*

1. In a pan over low heat, melt the olive oil, coconut oil, and beeswax.

2. Once melted, remove from heat, and add the essential oils. Stir to blend.

3. Pour into a 4-ounce mason jar, and put into the freezer for about 20 minutes to harden.

4. Apply with a gentle massage.

Makes 4 ounces

¼ cup olive oil

2 tablespoons unrefined
    coconut oil

2 tablespoons beeswax

20 drops lavender essential oil

20 drops ginger essential oil

15 drops frankincense
    essential oil

15 drops eucalyptus
    essential oil

Helpful Hint:
Arnica and St. John's Wort
are herbs well known for
their anti-inflammatory and
pain-relieving properties. For
an extra boost, steep 2 tablespoons of arnica flowers and
2 tablespoons of St. John's
Wort in the olive oil over low
heat for 2 hours. Strain, and
continue with the recipe.

Warming Circulation Massage Oil

Safe for ages 6+. Not safe for pregnant or
nursing mothers

*Cold hands and feet can hurt, especially if you experience
nerve pain. This blend helps to warm the body by improving
circulation, and it also aids in reducing spider veins.*

1. In a medium glass bowl, stir together the carrier oil
   and essential oils.

2. Pour the mixture into a lotion pump bottle (or preferred container).

3. Massage the oil into aching muscles, avoiding sensitive areas. Store in a cool, dark location.

Makes about 2 ounces

¼ cup carrier oil

15 drops ginger essential oil

10 drops black pepper
essential oil

10 drops cinnamon leaf
essential oil

5 drops clove bud essential oil

Helpful Hint: Naturally
anti-inflammatory and antispasmodic, cayenne pepper
contains a constituent called
capsaicin that is believed to
deplete neurotransmitters
that relay pain to the brain.
When cayenne is used
topically, it can help relieve
pain and increase circulation
where it's applied. To add the
warming benefits of cayenne
to this salve, steep 2 tablespoons of cayenne powder in
the carrier oil over low heat for
2 hours. Strain, and continue
with the recipe.

CHAPTER EIGHT:

For Personal Care

Minty Fresh Whitening Toothpaste

TOPICAL

Safe for ages 6+

I've been making toothpaste for nearly a decade, and my teeth couldn't be happier, healthier, or whiter. It's very easy to make your own toothpaste and tailor it to each person in your household. This recipe has activated charcoal and lemon essential oil to boost the natural white color of your teeth.

1. Using a hand mixer, mix coconut oil, baking soda, xylitol, and activated charcoal (if using) until a creamy paste is produced.

2. Add the essential oils, and mix until blended.

3. Squeeze a pea-size amount onto your toothbrush, and brush your teeth as usual.

Makes about 4 ounces

½ cup unrefined coconut oil (partially solidified)

¼ cup baking soda

¼ to ½ cup xylitol, finely ground

1 teaspoon activated charcoal (*optional*)

35 drops lemon essential oil

35 drops spearmint essential oil

Substitution Tip: Younger children tend to swallow some of their toothpaste while brushing, so this recipe is only for 6+ years of age. To make this toothpaste more kid-friendly, substitute 40 drops of strawberry flavor extract for the essential oils in this recipe.

Helpful Hint: Depending on the temperature, coconut oil may be more solid or liquid. Store your homemade toothpaste in a reusable squeeze bottle in a cool, dark location to ensure the best consistency.

Alcohol-Free Minty Mouthwash

TOPICAL

Safe for ages 6+. Not safe for pregnant or
nursing mothers

*Mouthwash, an important part of oral hygiene, helps
eliminate leftover bacteria and food that a toothbrush can't
reach. Alcohol-based mouthwash kills germs, but it also
dries out the mouth, which allows more bacteria to grow
and can cause other problems. I'm partial to alcohol-free
remedies like this one.*

1. Mix the water, hydrogen peroxide, and honey in a
   16-ounce amber glass bottle, and gently swirl until
   the honey is dissolved.

2. In a small glass bowl, mix the coconut oil and
   essential oils.

3. Add the oil mixture to the amber glass bottle, and
   seal shut.

4. Shake well to emulsify, and gargle with the mouthwash for 2 minutes. Do not swallow. Spit after
   gargling, and rinse mouth with water. Refrigerate
   when not in use.

Makes about 9 ounces

½ cup distilled water

½ cup hydrogen peroxide
(3 percent)

1 tablespoon raw
unfiltered honey

2 tablespoons fractionated
coconut oil

20 drops peppermint
essential oil

20 drops spearmint
essential oil

Substitution Tip: Pepper-
mint hydrosol, which can be
substituted for the filtered
water, is gentle and effective
as a mouthwash and has
a light minty flavor that is safe
for children. For a pregnancy/
kid-friendly toothpaste, use
peppermint hydrosol in place
of the water and omit the
coconut oil and essential oils
from the recipe.

Grapefruit Lavender Deodorant Paste

Makes about 8 ounces

¼ cup unrefined coconut oil

¼ cup shea butter

¼ cup arrowroot powder

1 tablespoon baking soda

3 tablespoons
   diatomaceous earth

16 drops grapefruit
   essential oil

16 drops lavender essential oil

It's easier than you might think to make your own natural and effective deodorant. I make mine like a whipped body butter—soft and easy to apply. You could add 2 tablespoons beeswax to this recipe and pour it into twist-up tubes if you prefer a deodorant stick.

1. In a pan over low heat, melt the coconut oil and shea butter.

2. While the coconut oil and shea butter are melting, mix the powders in a medium-size bowl.

3. Once melted, remove the coconut oil/shea butter mixture from the heat, and pour it into the powder mixture in the bowl.

4. Stir until the powders and oils are blended, and let the bowl cool in an ice bath.

5. Once the deodorant has cooled and hardened about halfway, use a hand mixer to whip the deodorant until it's a light and fluffy cream consistency.

6. While whipping the deodorant, add the essential oils, mixing them in.

7. Apply a pea-size amount of deodorant to your underarms, using your fingers to rub it in.

Peppermint Lavender Lip Balm

TOPICAL

Safe for ages 6+

Lip balm is an easy-to-make body care product and a big hit as a gift during the holiday season. It takes very few ingredients to create more than a dozen balms. The cooling effect of peppermint and healing properties of lavender help soothe and treat dry, chapped lips.

1. In a pan over low heat, melt the coconut oil, shea butter, and beeswax.
2. Once melted, remove from heat, and add the castor oil and essential oils. Stir to blend.
3. Pour the melted lip balm mixture into lip balm tubes, 0.5-ounce metal tins, or recycled mint tins, and let it cool and harden.
4. Apply to lips as a healing moisturizer.

Makes about 3 ounces

3 tablespoons unrefined coconut oil

1 tablespoon shea butter

1½ tablespoons beeswax

1 tablespoon castor oil

20 drops lavender essential oil

15 drops peppermint essential oil

Substitution Tip: For a kid-friendly lip balm option, substitute sweet orange essential oil for the peppermint essential oil in this recipe.

Helpful Hint: Pour lip balm into the empty half of a cute locket, and wear it around your neck.

Spiced Oranges and Honey Lip Scrub

TOPICAL

Makes about 2 ounces

Safe for ages 2+

Lip scrubs are great because they exfoliate dead skin while hydrating dry, chapped lips. This scrub relies on the humectant properties of both sugar and honey.

¼ cup sugar

1 tablespoon avocado oil

1 tablespoon raw
  unfiltered honey

1 teaspoon cinnamon powder

5 drops sweet orange
  essential oil

1. Mix all the ingredients in a small bowl, stirring to thoroughly combine.

2. Rub a small amount onto your lips in a circular motion for 1 to 2 minutes. Rinse off your lips with a warm, wet washcloth. Follow with an oil-based lip balm to lock in moisture.

Lemon Cookie Body Butter Bars

TOPICAL

Safe for ages 2+

Body butter is the most luxurious way to moisturize your skin, especially since water-based lotions evaporate much more quickly. These body butter bars are compact and great for travel.

1. In a pan over low heat, melt the coconut oil, shea butter, and beeswax.

2. Once melted, remove from heat, and add the essential oils. Stir to blend.

3. Pour the mixture into molds. For quick cooling, you can put them into the freezer for 20 minutes. Otherwise, these should sit on the counter to harden for 4 to 6 hours.

4. Once cooled and hardened, remove from the molds and store in a glass mason jar in a cool, dark location.

5. Melt the bar in the palms of your hand, and rub it all over your body for effective moisturizing with a delightful scent.

Makes about 6 ounces

¼ cup unrefined coconut oil

2 tablespoons shea butter

¼ cup beeswax

60 drops lemon essential oil (steam-distilled)

30 drops Roman chamomile essential oil

30 drops vanilla essential oil

Cooling Peppermint After-Sun Spray

TOPICAL

Safe for ages 6+

Summertime means outdoor fun, exercise, and sunshine, but it also can lead to heat exhaustion, sunburn, and dehydration. Peppermint essential oil can help when you've spent too much time outdoors and need to lower your body temperature or soothe reddened skin. For a pregnancy- and kid-friendly version, use spearmint essential oil instead of peppermint.

1. In an 8-ounce spray bottle, mix the aloe vera jelly, vegetable glycerin, and apple cider vinegar with the essential oils. Gently swirl to blend.
2. Add enough distilled water to fill the bottle.
3. Shake well and spray onto burned areas for relief. Cover your eyes before spraying the face.

Makes 8 ounces

¼ cup aloe vera jelly
½ tablespoon vegetable glycerin
1 tablespoon raw unfiltered apple cider vinegar
10 drops peppermint essential oil
10 drops lavender essential oil
Distilled water, to fill

Substitution Tip: Peppermint hydrosol is naturally anti-inflammatory and cooling to the skin. It can help clean and treat a burn while soothing the pain. Substitute peppermint hydrosol for the water in this recipe for an extra cooling after-sun spray.

Helpful Hint: Store this in the fridge for a super-cooled spray.

Peppermint Sage Facial Cleansing Grains

TOPICAL

Makes about 5 ounces

Safe for ages 6+

I don't wash my face with soap; I wash it with mud! Soap can be harsh, drying the skin and causing breakouts. Cleansing grains are a soap-free, exfoliating facial cleanser that naturally soothes inflamed skin, reduces fine lines, and heals acne and dermatitis. The best part of this recipe is that it doubles as a face mask.

¼ cup clay

2 tablespoons oats, finely ground

1 tablespoon coconut milk powder

2 tablespoons peppermint leaf, finely ground

2 tablespoons sage leaf, finely ground

8 drops peppermint essential oil

8 drops sage essential oil

1. Mix powdered ingredients in a bowl.

2. Add the essential oils. Using rubber or latex gloved hands, mix the essential oils into the powder until there are no clumps.

3. Store the cleansing grains in a spice jar with a shaker lid.

4. To use, mix up to 1 teaspoon of cleansing grains with a small amount of water or hydrosol in the palm of your hand. Apply the muddy mixture to your face, and gently scrub in a circular motion with your fingertips. Rinse with warm water, and follow with a toner and moisturizer.

Moisturizing Facial Toner

Safe for ages 2+

One of the most neglected steps in facial cleansing, toning helps remove excess oils and dead skin cells after washing. Toning also restores your face's pH, closes your pores, and helps moisturizer penetrate your skin better. This toner recipe is good for all skin types.

1. In a 4-ounce spray bottle, mix the witch hazel, aloe vera gel, and vegetable glycerin with the essential oils. Gently swirl to blend.
2. Add enough distilled water to fill the bottle.
3. Shake well, and spray onto a freshly cleaned face, avoiding contact with the eyes. Follow with a facial moisturizing oil.

Makes 4 ounces

¼ cup witch hazel
1 tablespoon aloe vera gel
1 teaspoon vegetable glycerin
5 drops lavender essential oil
3 drops grapefruit essential oil
3 drops coriander essential oil
Distilled water, to fill

Substitution Tip: Gentle and healing, rose hydrosol is great for all skin types and can be substituted for the water in this recipe.

Facial Moisturizing Oil

Safe for all ages

Whether you have oily or dry skin, you need a moisturizer to keep skin balanced, soft, and supple. I designed the carrier oil mixture for all skin types, and you can customize the essential oil blends based on your skin type listed here.

1. Mix carrier oils and essential oils in a 1-ounce pump top bottle. Gently swirl to blend.
2. After cleaning and toning your face, dispense 1 to 3 drops of moisturizing serum onto your palm, rub your hands together, and gently massage it onto your face. I use 1 drop of oil for my morning application and 2 or 3 drops of oil for my evening application.

Makes about 1 ounce

½ teaspoon hemp seed oil
½ teaspoon rosehip seed oil
½ teaspoon grapeseed oil
½ teaspoon pumpkin seed oil
Essential oils for your
    skin type

NORMAL SKIN TYPE

5 drops lavender essential oil
2 drops coriander essential oil

ACNE/OILY SKIN TYPE

3 drops geranium essential oil
3 drops grapefruit essential oil
1 drop rosalina essential oil

DRY/DAMAGED SKIN TYPE

2 drops Roman chamomile
    essential oil
2 drops coriander essential oil
3 drops sweet orange
    essential oil

MATURE SKIN TYPE

3 drops frankincense
    essential oil
2 drops rose essential oil
1 drop Roman chamomile
    essential oil

Detoxifying Facial Mask

Safe for ages 2+

My favorite girl's night event is a party I like to call Mudmask and Mimosas Monday. I invite all my girlfriends (and any men who want to participate) and tell them I'll provide luxurious mud masks if they bring the mimosas. This detoxifying mask is always a favorite.

1. Mix powdered ingredients in a bowl.

2. Add the essential oils. Using rubber or latex gloved hands, mix the essential oils into the powder until there are no clumps.

3. To use, mix 2 tablespoons of the blend with enough filtered water (or hydrosol, cooled herbal tea, or aloe vera gel) to create a paste.

4. Apply the herbal clay face mask to your face, avoiding hair, eyes, lips, and nostrils. Let it sit 15 to 20 minutes, misting with facial toner if it gets too itchy.

5. Rinse, and follow with facial toner and moisturizer. Store the powdered mixture in a mason jar.

Makes ½ cup

¼ cup bentonite clay
1 tablespoon activated charcoal
1 tablespoon lavender buds, finely ground
1 tablespoon dandelion leaf, finely ground
1 tablespoon green tea, finely ground
15 drops grapefruit essential oil
10 drops lemon essential oil
Distilled water

Citrus Fresh Moisturizing Body Wash

Body wash is one of my favorite ways to soap up in the shower. It's very easy to make, takes no time at all, and easily can be adapted to whatever ingredients you have on hand. Plus, this blend smells like a refreshing sunrise in your bathroom!

1. In a 16-ounce bottle with a flip-top lid, mix the Castile soap, vegetable glycerin, hemp seed oil, and essential oils. Seal tightly, and gently flip the bottle up and down to blend.

2. Squirt a quarter-size amount of body wash onto a loofah or washcloth, and rinse after washing.

Makes 16 ounces

1 cup liquid Castile soap

½ cup vegetable glycerin

½ cup hemp seed oil

50 drops sweet orange essential oil

50 drops grapefruit essential oil

20 drops bergamot essential oil

20 drops rosalina essential oil

Helpful Hint: For an extra moisturizing body wash, substitute 2 tablespoons of argan oil for 2 tablespoons of the hemp seed oil in this recipe.

Lavender Orange ACV Hair Conditioning Spray

Makes 16 ounces

Like the pores on your face, hair cuticles need to close after washing to give hair a healthy and shiny appearance. Soap often has a high pH, which opens cuticles. Closing them requires conditioner and a pH of between 4.5 and 5.5, which is closer to the sebum secreted by our skin. Apple cider vinegar is a well-known hair conditioner that can help reduce hair thinning, stimulate growth, and add strength and shine.

2 tablespoons raw unfiltered apple cider vinegar

2 tablespoons aloe vera jelly

10 drops lavender essential oil

10 drops sweet orange essential oil

Distilled water, to fill

1. Mix all the ingredients in a 16-ounce spray bottle.

2. Add water to fill.

3. Shake well, and spray onto wet hair. Gently comb through hair with your fingertips, and rinse with warm water.

Hair Growth Deep Conditioning Oil Treatment

TOPICAL

Safe for ages 6+

Many essential oils can improve your hair's luster, shine, and strength, but no other essential oil is quite as awesome as rosemary. When used in hair care products, rosemary essential oil reduces hair loss and increases hair growth, helping your mane grow to magical lengths.

Makes 1 treatment

1 teaspoon argan oil

1 teaspoon avocado oil

2 drops rosemary essential oil

2 drops Atlas cedarwood essential oil

1. In a small bowl, mix carrier oils and essential oils.

2. Apply to hair, working from the ends to the roots, and massage the oil into your scalp to promote hair growth.

3. Leave the conditioning oil treatment on hair for 1 to 2 hours before using shampoo.

4. Shampoo twice before conditioning. Repeat once a week to stimulate hair growth.

Detoxifying Hair and Scalp Mud Mask

TOPICAL

Safe for ages 2+

You can tell it's time for a detox when your hair feels weighted down by product buildup and your scalp produces more oils than usual. It's best to detoxify your hair and scalp once a month to help regulate oil production and improve luster.

1. In a medium-size bowl, thoroughly mix the bentonite clay, hemp seed oil, and essential oils.

2. Mix in the water 1 tablespoon at a time, until the blend is spreadable but not drippy.

3. Apply mixture to hair, cover with a shower cap to retain heat, and let sit for 15 minutes to an hour.

4. Rinse completely, and follow with an apple cider vinegar hair rinse.

Makes 1 treatment

¾ cup bentonite clay

1 tablespoon hemp seed oil

2 drops frankincense essential oil

2 drops sweet marjoram essential oil

2 to 6 tablespoons water, room temperature

Helpful Hint: This mud mask dries out hair the longer you leave it on, so it helps to spritz your hair with filtered water or hydrosol every so often. Try not to let the mask dry out.

Lavender Vanilla Ocean Waves Hair Spray

TOPICAL

Safe for all ages

If you want beachy hair when there's no ocean in sight, try making your own salty hair spray. This one combines the calming, floral aromas of lavender with the heady, intoxicating scents of vanilla, creating a scent and look that is irresistible.

Makes 8 ounces

½ cup distilled water, hot
2 tablespoons Epsom salt
1½ teaspoons sea salt
½ teaspoon hair conditioner
1 teaspoon vegetable glycerin
1 tablespoon aloe vera jelly
20 drops lavender essential oil
5 drops vanilla essential oil
Distilled water, to fill

1. Mix hot water, Epsom salt, sea salt, hair conditioner, and vegetable glycerin in a glass measuring cup. Stir until the salt is dissolved and the rest is mixed into the water.

2. In a small bowl, mix the aloe vera jelly and essential oils.

3. Using a funnel, add both mixtures to an 8-ounce spray bottle, and add water to fill.

4. Shake well, and spray onto wet or dry hair. Gently scrunch hair with your fingers, working from tips to roots, and either air-dry or blow-dry with a diffuser.

Easy Hair Pomade

TOPICAL

Safe for ages 2+

This simple pomade helps keep hair in place with a medium hold but can be made heavier by adding 2 more table-spoons of beeswax. Its conditioning and stimulating ingredients help improve hair quality, softness, and shine.

1. In a pan over low heat, melt the shea butter and beeswax.

2. Once melted, remove from heat, and add the arrow-root powder, hemp seed oil, and essential oils. Stir to blend.

3. Pour into an 8-ounce mason jar, and put into the freezer for about 20 minutes to harden.

4. Scoop out a pea-size amount, letting it melt between your palms before applying to hair. Style as usual.

Makes about 7 ounces

¼ cup plus 2 tablespoons shea butter

¼ cup beeswax

1 tablespoon arrowroot powder

¼ cup hemp seed oil

15 drops Atlas cedarwood essential oil

13 drops rosalina essential oil

5 drops fir needle essential oil

Soothing Shaving Cream

Safe for all ages

Making your own toiletries may seem like a daunting task, but many of your products share common ingredients. This recipe is made like whipped body butter, but it also contains liquid Castile soap and vegetable glycerin. This cream is perfect for legs, but I suggest omitting the Castile soap if you also plan to use it on your face because it can dry sensitive skin.

1. In a pan over low heat, melt the coconut oil and shea butter.
2. In a medium-size bowl, mix the liquid Castile soap and vegetable glycerin.
3. Add the hemp seed oil and clay to the soap mixture, and stir to blend.
4. Once the coconut oil and shea butter are melted, remove from heat and pour into the bowl with the other ingredients. Stir to blend.
5. Allow the shaving mixture to cool for a couple of hours.
6. Once the mixture is mostly firm, whip using your hand mixer until fluffy shaving cream is produced.
7. Add essential oils, and continue whipping for a few seconds longer to mix them in.
8. Squeeze shaving cream onto the palms of your hand, and rub onto skin. Follow with Razor Burn Aftershave Oil (see page 140) to keep skin soft, supple, and free of razor burn. Store in a reusable squeeze-top bottle in a cool, dark location to prevent melting.

Makes about
6 ounces whipped

¼ cup unrefined coconut oil

¼ cup shea butter

2 tablespoons liquid Castile soap

2 tablespoons vegetable glycerin

2 tablespoons hemp seed oil

1 tablespoon clay

20 drops lavender essential oil

10 drops Roman chamomile essential oil

Helpful Hint: Oils and butter can clog razors. Keep a cup of hot water with you in the shower to easily rinse off your razor between shaves.

Razor Burn Aftershave Oil

TOPICAL

Safe for ages 2+

Makes 2 ounces

The secret to avoiding razor burn, bumps, and inflamed skin is threefold: Exfoliate. Shave. Moisturize. This aftershave oil provides a soothing and healing moisturizer to combat any irritation.

2 tablespoons hemp seed oil

1 tablespoon pumpkin seed oil

1 tablespoon argan oil

20 drops sweet orange essential oil

15 drops rosalina essential oil

10 drops Roman chamomile essential oil

1. In a medium glass bowl, stir together the carrier oil and essential oils.

2. Pour the mixture into a lotion pump bottle (or preferred container).

3. Massage the oil into freshly shaven skin using about 1 or 2 drops for the face, 2 or 3 drops for the bikini area, and 5 or 6 drops per leg. Store in a cool, dark location.

Birthday Cake Sugar Scrub

TOPICAL

Safe for ages 2+

Makes about 8 ounces

Exfoliation is the key to soft, supple skin. Sugar scrubs are my favorite way to scrub away dead skin cells while restoring moisture. Every year on my birthday, I treat myself to this birthday cake sugar scrub. It softens rough skin and leaves a sweet scent.

1 cup sugar

¼ cup unrefined coconut oil, melted

Naturally colored sprinkles

20 drops vanilla essential oil

Substitution Tip: Out of sugar? This scrub also can be made with salt.

1. In a medium-size bowl, mix all the ingredients, stirring well.

2. Massage the scrub on skin, and rinse with hot water. (Caution, the tub may be slippery!) Store in a mason jar.

CHAPTER NINE:

For the Home

Orange Glass Cleaner

Safe for all ages

Cleaning your windows and mirrors can make a big difference in your home's appearance. This orange glass cleaner is easy to make and will clean glass surfaces without leaving streaks.

1. Mix ingredients in a 32-ounce spray bottle, and shake to blend.

2. Spray onto glass surface, and wipe clean using recycled newspaper, microfiber cloth, or paper towels.

Makes about 32 ounces

3 cups water

¼ cup plus 2 tablespoons rubbing alcohol

¼ cup plus 2 tablespoons distilled white vinegar

½ teaspoon sweet orange essential oil

Lemon Dusting Spray

CLEANING

Safe for all ages

Lemon essential oil cuts grease, disinfects, and leaves your home smelling of freshly squeezed lemons. This lemon dusting spray will clean and moisturize your wood surfaces.

1. In a 16-ounce spray bottle, mix olive oil, essential oil, and vinegar. Gently swirl to blend.

2. Add distilled water to fill the bottle.

3. Shake well, and spray onto wood surface. Wipe clean with a microfiber cloth.

Makes 16 ounces

2 teaspoons olive oil

¼ cup distilled white vinegar

20 drops lemon essential oil

Distilled water, to fill

All-Purpose Cleaner

CLEANING

Safe for all ages

This all-purpose cleaner relies on the high pH of Castile soap, borax, and washing soda to work its magic. (Avoid cleaning recipes that mix Castile soap and vinegar because the acidic nature of vinegar will cancel out the soap.) Both lavender and bergamot essential oils are naturally antiseptic and work to cut grease, lift stains, and disinfect surfaces.

1. Mix the hot water, washing soda, borax, and Castile soap in a bowl, stirring until dissolved.

2. Pour the mixture into a 16-ounce spray bottle, leaving enough room to add the essential oils. Add the oils, seal the bottle, and gently shake to blend.

Makes 16 ounces

2 cups water, hot

½ teaspoon washing soda

1 teaspoon borax

1 teaspoon liquid Castile soap

20 drops bergamot essential oil

10 drops lavender essential oil

Helpful Hint: Use this all-purpose cleaner for everything at home, from bathrooms to kitchens, carpets to floors—and even your car.

Lemon Pine Floor Mop Solution

CLEANING

Safe for all ages

Oxygen bleach is one of my favorite natural cleaning ingredients. It can whiten whites, deodorize garbage cans, and disinfect household surfaces. This mopping solution will clean the dirtiest of floors and leave your home with that classic lemon pine scent.

1. In a gallon-size bucket, stir together the oxygen bleach and essential oils.

2. Fill the bucket with hot water, and stir to dissolve the powder.

3. Mop floors.

Makes 1 treatment

1-gallon bucket

2 tablespoons oxygen bleach

20 drops lemon essential oil

20 drops pine essential oil

1 gallon hot water

Citrus Tea Tree Soft Scrub

Safe for all ages

I've used this soft scrub recipe for nearly a decade, and it's never failed me. It's highly antibacterial and antifungal, making it the perfect bathroom product to clean and whiten grout, tubs, toilets, and sinks. This soft scrub also is good at getting rid of mold, fungus, and other bacteria that lurk in damp areas.

1. In a large bowl, mix baking soda, Castile soap, water, and essential oils, stirring well to blend.

2. Scoop out what you need, and scrub it into surfaces using the scratchy side of a sponge. Store in a mason jar.

Makes about 3 cups

3 cups baking soda

½ cup liquid Castile soap

½ cup water

25 drops lemon essential oil

40 drops tea tree essential oil

½ teaspoon sweet orange essential oil

Helpful Hint: To whiten and brighten surfaces, spread the soft scrub on difficult-to-clean mold stains and grout. Let stand for 20 minutes, then rinse.

Orange Cedarwood Home and Garden Bug Spray

Safe for all ages

Summer weather means outdoor fun and gardening, but it also means bugs. This spray can be used both indoors and outdoors and on and around garden plants. This spray will kill all bugs, including the good ones like bees and butter-flies, so be mindful of where you use it. I have used it to kill ants, cockroaches, wasps, aphids, caterpillars, flies/horse-flies, and mosquitoes.

1. Mix ingredients in a 32-ounce spray bottle, and shake to blend.
2. Spray directly onto unwanted insects, or make this mixture in a large batch with boiling water to pour over ant colonies.

Makes 32 ounces

¼ cup liquid Castile soap

1 teaspoon sweet orange essential oil

1 teaspoon cedarwood essential oil

Distilled water, to fill

Carpet and Bed Refresher/Deodorizer

CLEANING

Safe for all ages

It's extremely easy and cost-effective to make your own baking soda carpet refresher. It takes only three ingredients and also can be used to freshen mattresses.

1. Mix baking soda and essential oils in a recycled spice jar, seal, and shake to incorporate the scent in the baking soda.
2. Sprinkle on carpets or mattresses, and let stand for 30 minutes before vacuuming up the powder.

Makes 1 cup

Baking soda, to fill

15 drops grapefruit essential oil

15 drops lavender essential oil

Substitution Tip: To give your mattress a calming bedtime scent, substitute Roman chamomile essential oil for grapefruit essential oil in this recipe.

Carpet and Upholstery Stain Remover

Safe for all ages

With five pets and one child, I've mastered the art of cleaning stains out of carpets and furniture. This blend uses the deodorizing powers of oxygen bleach, lemon, and rosalina to effectively remove stains from carpets, eradicate pet odors, and freshen fabrics.

Makes 1 treatment

2 cups hot water

2 teaspoons oxygen bleach

10 drops lemon essential oil

10 drops rosalina essential oil

1. Mix hot water and oxygen bleach in a bowl, and stir until dissolved.

2. Add the water mixture to a 16-ounce spray bottle, and add essential oils.

3. Shake well before use. Using the stream function on your spray bottle, spray carpet, upholstery, and clothing until stains are completely saturated. Allow to stand for 10 minutes before scrubbing clean. This also can be used in carpet steam cleaner vacuums.

Rosemary Bergamot Dish Soap

CLEANING

Safe ages 6+

I've tried many homemade dish soap recipes, and none impressed me. They either were too runny, combined vinegar and Castile soap (a no-no!), or didn't cut grease effectively. This dish soap is my cleaning glory! It sudses up just right, cuts grease, and cleans dishes without leaving any residue. Salt is important in this recipe to thicken the dish soap so it's not too watered down.

1. In a glass measuring cup, mix the warm water and salt, stirring until dissolved.

2. In a medium-size bowl, mix the Sal Suds, vinegar, and citric acid.

3. Slowly stir the salty water into the Sal Suds mixture until it thickens.

4. Stir in the essential oils, and pour into a recycled dish soap bottle.

Makes about 12 ounces

½ cup distilled water, warm

2 teaspoons salt

½ cup Dr. Bronner's Sal Suds

½ cup distilled white vinegar

1 teaspoon citric acid or lemon juice

10 drops rosemary essential oil

10 drops bergamot essential oil

Substitution Tip: For extra disinfectant power, substitute 20 drops of the Plague Killer Diffuser Blend (see page 73) for the essential oils in this recipe.

Lavender Lemon Dishwasher Powder

CLEANING

Safe for all ages

I've made liquid dishwasher soap and tablets, but nothing is as easy to whip up or works as well as this powder. Its combination of natural ingredients cleans stuck-on food and grease, and, just as important, dishes come out spot-free.

1. Mix powdered ingredients, stirring with a spoon.

2. Add essential oils, and stir until clumps disappear.

3. Use 1 to 2 tablespoons of powder per dish-washing cycle.

Makes 5 cups

2 cups washing soda

2 cups oxygen bleach

1 cup borax

20 drops lavender essential oil

20 drops lemon essential oil

Spring Fresh Fabric and Room Spray

CLEANING, AROMATIC

Safe for all ages

Makes 4 ounces

This spray brings a springtime freshness to your home. You also can use it on clothes, tossing them in the dryer for 10 minutes to refresh and de-wrinkle before wearing.

¼ cup witch hazel

60 drops grapefruit essential oil

60 drops bergamot essential oil

30 drops coriander essential oil

30 drops rosalina essential oil

Distilled water, to fill

1. In a 4-ounce spray bottle, mix witch hazel with the essential oils. Gently swirl to blend.

2. Add distilled water to fill the bottle.

3. Shake well, and spray into the air and on furniture and bedding (pillows, blankets, sheets, mattresses, and bedroom curtains). Store in a cool, dark location.

Euca-Citru-Licious Poo-Pourri Spray

CLEANING, AROMATIC

Safe for ages 6+

Makes 4 ounces

The magic behind this spray is that it creates an essential oil layer on top of toilet water before use. The protective barrier traps odors under the surface, so no more embarrassing smells!

25 drops eucalyptus essential oil

25 drops lemon essential oil

25 drops bergamot essential oil

25 drops grapefruit essential oil

Witch hazel, to fill

1. Add essential oils to a 4-ounce spray bottle. Gently swirl to blend.

2. Add witch hazel to fill the bottle, and seal with the lid.

3. Before using the toilet, shake well and spray into the toilet bowl 8 to 10 times. The essential oils will disperse over the water, creating a protective scent barrier. Store in a cool, dark location.

Helpful Hint: Keep a bottle in your purse or backpack, and use it in public restrooms and the office.

Citrus Fresh Garbage Disposal Deodorizer

CLEANING

Safe for all ages

Citrus fruit peels contain essential oils, so they often are cold-pressed instead of steam-distilled. You can use these peels as a simple and cost-effective way to clean and deodorize the garbage disposal in your kitchen sink.

With sink water running, toss a few pieces into the garbage disposal while it's turned on.

Makes 1 treatment

Fresh lemon peels, torn into
  1-inch pieces

Substitution Tip: All citrus peels carry the essential oils of their fruit. You can substitute any citrus peels for the lemon peels in this recipe.

Trash Can Deodorizer Tablets

CLEANING

Safe for all ages

Baking soda is a natural cleaning favorite when it comes to deodorizing the home. When combined with the refreshing scents of lemongrass and lavender, these tablets guarantee your trash can will never smell the same again.

1. Wearing rubber or latex gloves, mix the baking soda and essential oils in a medium-size bowl, breaking up any clumps with your fingers.

2. Add water to the mixture 1 tablespoon at a time, and continue to mix using your gloved hands until it packs together (like a snowball) without crumbling.

3. Tightly pack the mixture into silicone molds or mini muffin tins, and leave overnight to dry and harden.

4. Leave one tablet in the bottom of a trash can before inserting a new bag. Replace tablets once a week.

Makes 6 to 8 tablets

1 cup baking soda

10 drops lemongrass
  essential oil

20 drops lavender essential oil

4 tablespoons water

¼-cup silicone molds or mini
  muffin tin

Upholstery Cleaner

Safe for all ages

I once bought cream-colored dining room chairs while my son was still a toddler. After our first meal, a spaghetti dinner, I instantly realized I had made a mistake. That's when I came up with this recipe for a natural upholstery cleaner. It worked miracles, returning my red sauce–splattered chairs to their former glory.

Makes 16 ounces

2 cups distilled water

2 tablespoons liquid
  Castile soap

2 tablespoons washing soda

25 drops sweet marjoram
  essential oil

25 drops lemon essential oil

1. In a glass measuring cup, mix water, Castile soap, and washing soda, stirring until dissolved.

2. Add the soap mixture and essential oils to a 16-ounce spray bottle. Seal with the lid, and shake to emulsify.

3. Spray stains on upholstery, and let stand for 30 minutes before scrubbing clean with a dry washcloth or sponge.

Citronella Cedarwood Candles

AROMATIC

Safe for all ages

Citronella candles keep mosquitoes away while you're enjoying summer in your backyard. These DIY candles are very easy and cost-effective. Pour the wax mixture into metal tins instead of glass jars for outdoor-friendly bug repellent candles. Take them camping, on picnics, or to the beach.

1. In a pan over low heat, melt the soy wax and beeswax.
2. Once melted, remove from heat, and add essential oils.
3. Place the candle wick into your chosen container.
4. Pour the mixture into the candle jars, and let them cool and harden.

Makes 16 ounces

1 cup soy wax flakes

1 cup beeswax

100 drops citronella
  essential oil

80 drops cedarwood
  essential oil

Candle wicks

Recycled candle jars or
  metal tins

Helpful Hint: While the wax is cooling, place a butter knife flat across the top of the candle jar to hold the wick in place until the wax hardens.

Clean Linen Laundry Powder

There are many ways to make your own laundry soap, but this recipe is designed for busy people who don't have time to melt ingredients every time they need a new batch. This laundry powder also is safe for high-efficiency machines and can be used to clean cloth diapers.

1. In a large bowl, mix powdered ingredients with a whisk.

2. Add essential oils, and continue stirring until there are no clumps.

3. Use ¼ cup of laundry powder per load. Store in an airtight container in your laundry room.

Makes 8 cups

1 cup soap flakes

1 cup oxygen bleach

3 cups washing soda

1 cup borax

2 cups baking soda

40 drops grapefruit essential oil

40 drops rosalina essential oil

Helpful Hint: For extra soft clothes, add 1 cup of ice cream salt to this recipe. Distilled white vinegar, which also can be added as a fabric softener, rinses out and won't leave your clothes smelling like vinegar.

Homemade Bleach Alternative

CLEANING

Safe for all ages

When I decided to get rid of toxic cleaning products in my home, bleach was the first to go because it can cause all sorts of health issues after repeated use. This homemade bleach alternative does everything that bleach can do without its toxic fumes.

1. Mix peroxide, lemon juice, citric acid, and essential oil in a ½-gallon amber glass jug.

2. Add water to fill. Seal with the lid, and gently shake jug to blend.

3. Shake the bottle before use, and use as you would bleach: in your laundry to whiten whites, in your bathroom and kitchen to disinfect, and in your dishwasher as a rinse aid. Store in a cool, dark location.

Makes ½ gallon

¾ cup hydrogen peroxide
(3 percent)
¼ cup lemon juice
1 tablespoon citric acid
20 drops lemon essential oil
Distilled water, to fill

Lavender Dreams "Dryer Sheets"

AROMATIC

Safe for all ages

Essential oils can give your laundry that fresh-from-the-dryer smell. These homemade "dryer sheets" are not only cost-effective but also are environmentally friendly.

Add essential oil drops to the damp washcloth, and toss it into the laundry for the last 10 minutes of the drying cycle.

Makes 1 treatment

1 clean, damp washcloth
5 drops lavender essential oil
3 drops vanilla essential oil

Lemon Furniture Polish

CLEANING

Safe for all ages

It may be my Greek heritage, but I've always used olive oil in multiple ways throughout my home. This lemon furniture polish will clean and condition your wood furniture, leaving behind a lovely, fresh scent.

1. Whip together coconut oil and olive oil using a fork.

2. Stir in the essential oil.

3. Using a small amount, buff wood furniture in a circular motion with a microfiber cloth until it shines.

Makes 4 ounces

2 tablespoons unrefined coconut oil

12 drops olive oil

9 drops lemon essential oil

Substitution Tip: Jojoba oil is not an oil. It's actually a liquid wax that works well on wood furniture and floors and can be substituted for the olive oil in this recipe.

Glossary

ANALGESIC: relieves pain

ANTIBACTERIAL: fights the growth of bacteria

ANTIDEPRESSANT: helps counteract depression and lifts the mood

ANTIFUNGAL: prevents the growth of fungi

ANTI-INFLAMMATORY: reduces inflammation and swelling

ANTISEPTIC: prevents the spread of bacteria and viruses

ANTISPASMODIC: relieves muscle spasms

ANTITUSSIVE: prevents and relieves coughs

ASTRINGENT: shrinks or constricts the skin

CARMINATIVE: helps relieve gas, stomach pains, and digestive issues

CICATRIZANT: scar healing

DEPURATIVE: detoxifying

DIAPHORETIC: induces sweating

DIURETIC: promotes excretion of water from the body

EMMENAGOGUE: stimulates menstrual flow

EXPECTORANT: helps rid the lungs of phlegm and mucus

FEBRIFUGE: reduces fevers

NERVINE: calms the nerves

SEDATIVE: promotes calming and sleep

VULNERARY: heals wounds

Travel Kit

Traveling takes a toll on everyone, but a carefully planned essential oil travel kit can make the difference between a good trip and a bad one. Many of the recipes in this book are portable when placed in travel-size containers (be sure to check airline carry-on regulations), including the roll-ons, personal inhalers, and healing salve recipes. I always pack a couple of my favorite essential oils in ½-ounce bottles in my travel kit. With so many uses, I never know when I might need one!

Lavender Essential Oil: Lavender is versatile for traveling. Inhaling it can calm jitters, soothe anxiety, and help relax your mind and body for sleep. Naturally antiseptic, a couple of drops of lavender can clean and treat wounds when diluted in aloe vera jelly or fractionated coconut oil. Dilute 6 to 8 drops and add to your hotel bath for a better night's rest. Add a couple of drops to your camping chairs to repel mosquitoes.

Peppermint Essential Oil: Motion sickness, headaches, and grogginess all can be remedied with a whiff of peppermint. Dilute 2 drops and apply to bug bites to relieve itching. Add a drop to a tissue placed in an air-conditioning vent to diffuse the oil in your car. Dilute 5 drops of peppermint, 5 drops of lavender, and 5 drops of rosalina essential oils per ounce (2 tablespoons) of coconut oil for an on-the-go vapor rub.

Rosalina Essential Oil: Referred to as "lavender tea tree," rosalina can do the work of lavender, tea tree, and eucalyptus essential oils. It can clean germs in an antibacterial hand blend if you mix 9 drops of rosalina per ounce (2 tablespoons) of aloe vera jelly. Naturally antiseptic and anti-inflammatory, rosalina also can clean and treat wounds, spot treat acne, and soothe stiff muscles when diluted. To freshen stale air in the car, add a drop to a tissue and place it in an air-conditioning vent.

Fractionated Coconut Oil: I always carry a 3.4-ounce bottle to dilute essential oils for topical use. It also can be used as a base for massage oils, aromatherapy roll-ons, quick baths, soothing moisturizers, and skin ointments.

Aloe Vera Jelly: I always carry a 3.4-ounce bottle of this, too. Water soluble with a quick absorption rate, aloe vera jelly is aloe vera gel mixed with an emulsifier, allowing you to easily dilute essential oils with water for hand and facial gels, quick baths, nongreasy moisturizing, and itch relief.

Resources

If you are just starting out on your aromatherapy journey, many great resources are available for you to find aromatherapy schools or an aromatherapist and to purchase essential oils. Here are some of my favorite resources to help you get more out of essential oils.

Alliance of International Aromatherapists (www.Alliance-Aromatherapists.org)

This nonprofit alliance seeks to advance aromatherapy research, promote the responsible use of essential oils, and establish and maintain professional educational standards.

Anthis, Christina. *The Complete Book of Essential Oils for Mama and Baby: Safe and Natural Remedies for Pregnancy, Birth, and Children.* Emeryville: Althea Press, 2017.

If you or someone you know is pregnant or nursing, or has children, my book is full of recipes and information on the safe use of essential oils at every age.

Mountain Rose Herbs (www.MountainRoseHerbs.com)

Mountain Rose Herbs is an eco-friendly source for 100-percent certified organic herbs, essential oils, carrier oils, and other ingredients needed to make personal care items and cosmetics.

National Association For Holistic Aromatherapy (NAHA.org)

This member-based nonprofit association provides a wealth of aromatherapy knowledge, including scientific information, safety data, education resources, professional standards, and a list of certified aromatherapists.

Plant Therapy Essential Oils (www.PlantTherapy.com)

One of my favorite sources for all things essential oils, Plant Therapy is an affordable source for high-quality essential oils, carrier oils, and aromatherapy accessories. The company worked with Robert Tisserand to create KidSafe® sets of essential oil blends.

Tisserand, Robert, and Rodney Young. *Essential Oil Safety: A Guide for Health, 2nd Edition.* Philadelphia: Churchill Livingstone, 2013.

This is an updated and comprehensive book on safety standards for essential oils. It contains chemical profiles, as well as safety data and recommendations.

References

Alliance of International Aromatherapists. "Aromatherapy." Accessed April 20, 2019. www.alliance-aromatherapists.org/aromatherapy.

Bauer, Brent. "What Are the Benefits of Aromatherapy?" *Mayo Clinic Consumer Health.* Accessed April 22, 2019. www.mayoclinic.org/healthy-lifestyle/consumer-health /expert-answers/aromatherapy/faq-20058566.

Ben-Arye, E., N. Dudai, A. Eini, M. Torem, E. Schiff, and Y. Rakover. "Treatment of Upper Respiratory Tract Infections in Primary Care: A Randomized Study Using Aromatic Herbs." *Evidence-Based Complementary and Alternative Medicine* 2011, no. 690346 (2011): 7 pages. doi.org/10.1155/2011/690346.

Bensouilah, Janetta, and Philippa Buck. *Aromadermatology: Aromatherapy in the Treatment and Care of Common Skin Conditions.* Routledge, 2001. Kindle edition.

Berdejo, D., B. Chueca, E. Pagán, A. Renzoni, W.L. Kelley, R. Pagán, and D. Garcia-Gonzalo. "Sub-Inhibitory Doses of Individual Constituents of Essential Oils Can Select for *Staphylococcus aureus* Resistant Mutants." *Molecules* 24, no. 1 (January 2019): 170. doi:10.3390/molecules24010170.

Borges, A., A. Abreu, C. Dias, M.J. Saavedra, F. Borges, and M. Simões. "New Perspectives on the Use of Phytochemicals as an Emergent Strategy to Control Bacterial Infections Including Biofilms." *Molecules* 21, no. 7 (July 2016): 877. doi:10.3390 /molecules21070877.

Buckle, Jane. *Clinical Aromatherapy: Essential Oils in Healthcare.* 3rd ed. Philadelphia: Churchill Livingstone, 2014.

Catty, Suzanne. *Hydrosols: The Next Aromatherapy.* Rochester: Healing Arts Press, 2001.

Choi, S., P. Kang, H. Lee, and G. Seol. "Effects of Inhalation of Essential Oil of *Citrus aurantium* L. var. *amara* on Menopausal Symptoms, Stress, and Estrogen in Postmenopausal Women: A Randomized Controlled Trial." *Evidence-Based Complementary and Alternative Medicine* 2014, no. 796518 (2014): 7 pages. doi: 10.1155/2014/796518.

Clark, Demetria. *Aromatherapy and Herbal Remedies for Pregnancy, Birth, and Breast-feeding.* Summertown: Healthy Living Publications, 2015.

Clark, Marge. *Essential Oils and Aromatics: A Step-by-Step Guide for Use in Massage and Aromatherapy.* Amazon Digital Services LLC, 2013. Kindle edition.

de Aguiar, F.C., A.L. Solarte, C. Tarradas, I. Luque, A. Maldonado, Á. Galán-Relaño, and B. Huerta. "Antimicrobial Activity of Selected Essential Oils Against *Streptococcus suis* Isolated from Pigs." *MicrobiologyOpen* 7, no. 6 (March 2018): 6 pages. doi:10.1002/mbo3.613.

Deckard, Angela. "11 Proven Peppermint Essential Oil Benefits." *Healthy Focus*. Accessed April 21, 2019. healthyfocus.org/proven-peppermint-essential-oil-benefits.

Dennerlein, Roseann. "What Is a Clinical Aromatherapist?" *Oils of Shakan*. Accessed April 22, 2019. oilsofshakan.com/what-is-a-clinical-aromatherapist/.

Environmental Working Group. "Toxic Cleaner Fumes Could Contaminate California Classrooms." *Press Release*. Accessed April 22, 2019. www.ewg.org/news/news-releases/2009/10/28/toxic-cleaner-fumes-could-contaminate-california-classrooms.

Fifi, A.C., C.H. Axelrod, P. Chakraborty, and M. Saps. "Herbs and Spices in the Treatment of Functional Gastrointestinal Disorders: A Review of Clinical Trials." *Nutrients* 10, no. 11 (November 2018): 1715. doi:10.3390/nu10111715.

Furlow, F. "The Smell of Love." *Psychology Today*. Accessed April 22, 2019. www.psychologytoday.com/us/articles/199603/the-smell-love.

Gattefossé, René-Maurice. *Gattefossé's Aromatherapy: The First Book on Aromatherapy*. 2nd ed. London: Ebury Digital, 2012. Kindle edition.

Gatti, Giovanni, and Renato Cajola. *The Action of Essences on the Nervous System*. Italy: 1923.

Hinton, D.E., T. Pham, M. Tran, S.A. Safren, M.W. Otto, and M.H. Pollack. "CBT for Vietnamese Refugees with Treatment-Resistant PTSD and Panic Attacks: A Pilot Study." *Journal of Traumatic Stress* 17, no. 5 (October 2004): 429–33. doi:10.1023/B:JOTS.0000048956.03529.fa.

Hirsch, A., and J. Gruss. "Human Male Sexual Response to Olfactory Stimuli." *American Academy of Neurological and Orthopaedic Surgeons*. Accessed on April 22, 2019. aanos.org/human-male-sexual-response-to-olfactory-stimuli/.

Hüsnü Can Baser, K., and Gerhad Buchbauer. *Handbook of Essential Oils: Science, Technology, and Applications*. 2nd ed. Boca Raton: CRC Press, 2015.

Inouye, Shigeharu, Toshio Takizawa, and Hideyo Yamaguchi. "Antibacterial Activity of Essential Oils and Their Major Constituents Against Respiratory Tract Pathogens by Gaseous Contact." *Journal of Antimicrobial Chemotherapy* 47, no. 5 (May 2001): 565–73. doi:10.1093/jac.47.5.565.

Keim, Joni, and Ruah Bull. *Aromatherapy & Subtle Energy Techniques: Compassionate Healing with Essential Oils.* CreateSpace, 2015.

Khadivzadeh, T., M. Najafi, M. Ghazanfarpour, M. Irani, F. Dizavandi, F. and K. Shariati. "Aromatherapy for Sexual Problems in Menopausal Women: A Systematic Review and Meta-analysis." *Journal of Menopausal Medicine* 24, no. 1 (April 2018): 56–61. doi:10.6118/jmm.2018.24.1.56.

Kline, R.M., J.J. Kline, J. Di Palma, and G.J. Barbero. "Enteric-Coated, Ph-Dependent Peppermint Oil Capsules for the Treatment of Irritable Bowel Syndrome in Children." *Journal of Pediatrics* 138, no. 1 (January 2001): 125–8. www.ncbi.nlm.nih.gov/pubmed/11148527.

Knezevic, P., V. Aleksic, N. Simin, E. Svircev, A. Petrovic, and N. Mimica-Dukic. "Antimicrobial Activity of *Eucalyptus camaldulensis* Essential Oils and Their Interactions with Conventional Antimicrobial Agents Against Multi-Drug Resistant *Acinetobacter baumannii*." *Journal of Ethnopharmacology* 178 (February 2016): 125–36. doi:10.1016/j.jep.2015.12.008.

Köse, E., M. Sarsilmaz, S. Meydan, M. Sönmez, M., I. Kus, and A. Kavakli. "The Effect of Lavender Oil on Serum Testosterone Levels and Epididymal Sperm Characteristics of Formaldehyde Treated Male Rats." *European Review for Medical and Pharmacological Sciences* 15, no. 5 (May 2011): 538–42. www.ncbi.nlm.nih.gov/pubmed/21744749.

Koulivand, P.H., M. Khaleghi Ghadiri, and A. Gorji. "Lavender and the Nervous System." *Evidence-Based Complementary and Alternative Medicine* 2013, no. 681304 (2013): 10 pages. doi:10.1155/2013/681304.

Lafata, Alexia. "How Our Sense of Smell Makes Us Fall In Love and Stay in Love." *Elite Daily*. Accessed April 22, 2019. www.elitedaily.com/dating/sense-of-smell-makes-us-love/1094795.

Lahmar, A., A. Bedoui, I. Mokdad-Bzeouich, Z. Dhaouifi, Z. Kalboussi, I. Cheraif, K. Ghedira, and L. Chekir-Ghedira. "Reversal of Resistance in Bacteria Underlies Synergistic Effect of Essential Oils with Conventional Antibiotics." *Microbial Pathogenesis* 106 (May 2017): 50–9. doi:10.1016/j.micpath.2016.10.018.

Lawless, Julia. *The Encyclopedia of Essential Oils: The Complete Guide to the Use of Aromatic Oils in Aromatherapy, Herbalism, Health & Well-Being.* Berkeley: Conari Press, 2013.

Lee, K., E. Cho, and Y. Kang. "Changes in 5-Hydroxytryptamine and Cortisol Plasma Levels in Menopausal Women After Inhalation of Clary Sage Oil." *Phytotherapy Research* 28, no. 12 (December 2014): 1599–1605. doi:10.1002/ptr.5163.

Lillehei, A.S., and L.L. Halcon. "A Systematic Review of the Effect of Inhaled Essential Oils on Sleep." *Journal of Alternative and Complementary Medicine* 20, no. 6 (June 2014): 441–51. doi:10.1089/acm.2013.0311.

Mojay, G. *Aromatherapy for Healing the Spirit: A Guide to Restoring Emotional and Mental Balance Through Essential Oils.* London: Gardners Books, 2005.

Morris, Edwin. *Scents of Time: Perfume from Ancient Egypt to the 21st Century.* New York: The Metropolitan Museum of Art, 1999.

Nagai, K., A. Niijima, Y. Horii, J. Shen, and M. Tanida "Olfactory Stimulatory with Grapefruit and Lavender Oils Change Autonomic Nerve Activity and Physiological Function." *Autonomic Neuroscience* 185 (June 2014): 29–35. doi:10.1016/j.autneu.2014.06.005.

National Association for Holistic Aromatherapy. "Safety Information." Accessed April 23, 2019. naha.org/explore-aromatherapy/safety.

Ostling, Michael. "Witches' Herbs on Trial." *Folklore* 125, no. 2 (July 2014): 179–201. doi:10.1080/0015587X.2014.890785.

Pertz, H., J. Lehmann, R. Roth-Ehrang, and S. Elz. "Effects of Ginger Constituents on the Gastrointestinal Tract: Role of Cholinergic M3 and Serotonergic 5-HT3 and 5-HT4 receptors." *Planta Medica* 77, no. 10 (July 2011): 973–8. doi:10.1055/s-0030-1270747.

Prabuseenivasan, Seenivasan, Manickkam Jayakumar, and Savarimuthu Ignacimuthu. "*In Vitro* Antibacterial Activity of Some Plant Essential Oils." *BMC Complementary and Alternative Medicine* 6, no. 39 (November 2006): 196–207. doi:10.1186/1472-6882-6-39.

Price, Shirley. *Aromatherapy Workbook: A Complete Guide to Understanding and Using Essential Oils.* Amazon Digital Services LLC, 2012. Kindle edition.

Raho, Bachir, and M. Benali. "Antibacterial Activity of the Essential Oils from the Leaves of *Eucalyptus globulus* Against *Escherichia coli* and *Staphylococcus aureus*." *Asian Pacific Journal of Tropical Biomedicine* 2, no. 9 (September 2012): 739–42. doi:10.1016/S2221-1691(12)60220-2.

Rose, J., and F. Behm. "Inhalation of Vapor from Black Pepper Extract Reduces Smoking Withdrawal Symptoms." *Drug and Alcohol Dependence* 34, no. 3 (February 1994): 225–9. doi:10.1016/0376-8716(94)90160-0.

Schnaubelt, Kurt. *The Healing Intelligence of Essential Oils: The Science of Advanced Aromatherapy*. Rochester: Healing Arts Press, 2011.

Sienkiewicz, M., A. Głowacka, E. Kowalczyk, A. Wiktorowska-Owczarek, M. Jóźwiak-Bębenista, and M. Łysakowska. "The Biological Activities of Cinnamon, Geranium and Lavender Essential Oils." *Molecules* 19, no. 12 (December 2014): 20929–40. doi:10.3390/molecules191220929.

Silva, G.L., C. Luft, A. Lunardelli, R.H. Amaral, D.A. Melo, M.V. Donadio, F.B. Nunes, et al. "Antioxidant, Analgesic and Anti-Inflammatory Effects of Lavender Essential Oil." *Anais da Academia Brasileira de Ciências* 87, no. 2 (August 2015): 1397–1408. doi:10.1590/0001-3765201520150056.

Srivastava, J.K., E. Shankar, and S. Gupta. "Chamomile: A Herbal Medicine of the Past with a Bright Future." *Molecular Medicine Reports* 3 (September 2010): 895–901. doi:10.3892/mmr.2010.377.

Stea, Susanna, Alina Beraudi, and Dalila De Pasquale. "Essential Oils for Complementary Treatment of Surgical Patients: State of the Art." *Evidence-Based Complementary and Alternative Medicine* 2014, no. 726341 (February 2014): 6 pages. doi:10.1155/2014/726341.

Valnet, Jean. *The Practice of Aromatherapy: A Classic Compendium of Plant Medicines and Their Healing Properties*. London: Ebury Digital, 2012. Kindle edition.

WebMD. "Growing Pains." Accessed April 22, 2019. www.webmd.com/children/guide/growing-pains#1.

Worwood, Valerie Ann. *Aromatherapy for the Healthy Child: More Than 300 Natural, Nontoxic, and Fragrant Essential Oil Blends*. Amazon Digital Services LLC, 2012. Kindle edition.

Worwood, Valerie Ann. *The Fragrant Mind: Aromatherapy for Personality, Mind, Mood, and Emotion*. London: Ebury Digital, 2012. Kindle edition.

Worwood, Valerie Ann. *Scents & Scentuality: Essential Oils & Aromatherapy for Romance, Love, and Sex*. Amazon Digital Services LLC: New World Library, 2012. Kindle edition.

Yap, P.S., B.C. Yiap, H.C. Ping, and S.H. Lim. "Essential Oils, A New Horizon in Combating Bacterial Antibiotic Resistance." *The Open Microbiology Journal* 8 (February 2014): 6–14. doi:10.2174/1874285801408010006.

Yap, P.S., S.H. Lim, and B.C. Yiap. "Combination of Essential Oils and Antibiotics Reduce Antibiotic Resistance in Plasmid-Conferred Multidrug Resistant Bacteria." *Phytomedicine* 20, no. 8–9 (June 2013): 710–3. doi:10.1016/j.phymed.2013 .02.013.

Yavari Kia, P., F. Safajou, M. Shahnazi, and H. Nazemiyeh. "The Effect of Lemon Inhalation Aromatherapy on Nausea and Vomiting of Pregnancy: A Double-Blinded, Randomized, Controlled Clinical Trial." *Iranian Red Crescent Medical Journal* 16, no. 3 (March 2014): e14360. doi:10.5812/ircmj.14360.

Zainol, N.A., T.S. Ming, and Y. Darwis. "Development and Characterization of Cinnamon Leaf Oil Nanocream for Topical Application." *Indian Journal of Pharmaceutical Sciences* 77, no. 4 (July–August 2015): 422–33. www.ncbi.nlm .nih.gov/pubmed/26664058.

Recipe Index

Ailment Index

General Index

Acknowledgments

Writing a book is a hefty task, and I couldn't have done it without the love and support of so many people in my life. I would like to thank my son, Silas, for being my miracle and loving me every single day. Clint Hill, I couldn't have written this book without you. I'd like to thank you for listening to me rattle on about essential oils every single day for a month, for still kissing me on all the days I didn't shower, and for your constant belief in me and my abilities. I would really like to thank my mom and dad for their constant, undying support in all things that I pursue. Without you guys, I may never have become a writer. Thank you for giving me the tools I've needed to follow my own path and think outside of the box. Mom, you introduced me to the wonderful world of writing, and Dad, you taught me how to look at the world from an engineer's perspective. Finally, I would not have a book without all the wonderful people at Callisto who worked really hard to make this book happen. Vanessa Ta, you are a rock star editor, and without your support and tireless efforts, I might never have finished this book!

About the Author

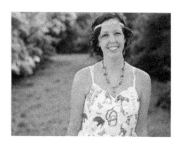

CHRISTINA ANTHIS is a single mother and the blogger behind *The Hippy Homemaker*. As a committed do-it-yourselfer trained in aromatherapy and herbalism, she is devoted to helping others make safe and natural health and home-care products with essential oils. Christina, her son, and her partner, Clint, make their home in Texas.